SELF-CARE RX

A Doctor's Guide to Transformation After Trauma

Danielle DonDiego, DO, MBA

Copyright © 2021 by Danielle DonDiego, DO, MBA

Book Design and Interior by Damonza

All rights reserved. This book or any portion thereof may not be reproduced or used in any manner whatsoever without the express written permission of the publisher except for the use of brief quotations in a book review.

Printed in the United States of America

First Printing, 2021

ISBN (paperback) 978-1-7371807-0-8

eBook ISBN 978-1-7371807-1-5

ACKNOWLEDGEMENTS

To say this has been a wild journey is an understatement. It is not lost on me that I am where I am because I've found people who have shown unconditional love and support through all of this.

I want to thank those that contributed their stories to this book: Dawn, Karla, Diana and Joanna. It is empowering to witness everyone share their stories as raw and real as they are. It takes a lot of courage to share, thank you for your bravery.

I want to thank my friends that have spent hours on the phone with me, let me cry, traveled with me, given me places to stay, food, and dealt with my life transition without judgment.

I want to thank my family for doing their best with the situations at hand, good and bad.

I want to thank those in my residency program who covered for me when I needed it and looked out for me while completing training. There are plenty of moments I never verbalized that I recognized your help or grace and I want to acknowledge that I saw those moments more than I ever spoke out loud.

My therapist is an absolute rock star, and honestly was the first person to really help me look at what the hell was going on in my life and who I really am—thank you isn't enough. :)

Candi, thank you for your patience with this project and incredible ability to transmit this story in a way that the world can benefit from.

Geno, my amazing pup who has been my buddy for the last ten years and dealt with lots of moves and new places.

Lastly, I want to acknowledge all survivors who are currently healing or may be going through something horrific. You are not alone, not by a long shot. Surround yourself with people that bring you joy, and it'll be easier to gain the strength to make the hard decisions when you're ready. You will know when it's best to take action, trust yourself over anyone else.

INTRODUCTION
Extreme Strength Training

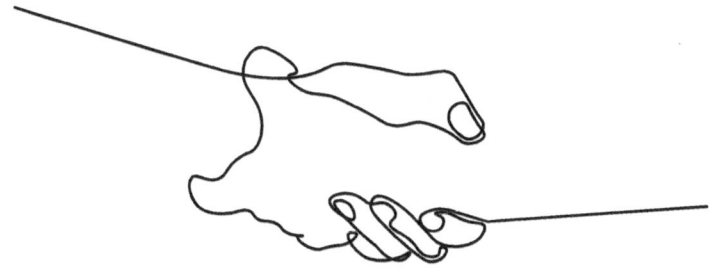

> "Personal transformation can and does have global effects. As we go, so goes the world, for the world is us. The revolution that will save the world is ultimately a personal one."
>
> —Marianne Williamson

Self-Care RX

THINK OF THE most beautiful flower in the world. It may be a red rose, blue hydrangea, cherry blossom, yellow gardenia, or sunflower. What if you could feel that beautiful, light, captivating, and strong in your presence inside out every day?

Your self-care can result in this. That very magnetism and spectacular vibrancy must be cultivated inside first. The inside is defined by your mental state, relationship with yourself and others, purpose, fulfillment, boundaries, perseverance, self-talk, beliefs, and discernment. Once these components are solid within your existence, your physical appearance may be much easier to solidify how you desire it to be.

One of my favorite flowers is the eye-catching protea, which is known to symbolize change and transformation.

After years of therapy, personal development, and other transformational tools, along with trying areligious forms of spirituality over the last several years, I look back on the first thirty years of my life and feel that version of me has died. When you go through trauma and decide to take the journey of healing rather than self-destruction, it's common to have some level of an existential crisis. I'd say mine slowly dripped out over time. Going from a human bred for achievement based on social constructs of accomplishment, to realizing I am simply a soul in a human's body having an experience on earth, I have become an entirely new version of myself. This version will evolve as long as I continue to put forth the effort.

Self-care has many layers. The most superficial of them being spa days, bubble baths, and the like. The deepest layer of self-care being full commitment to self-discovery, evolution, and a nonnegotiable respect for self. I've been through every layer, ignored all of them, and now honor each of them. You can't take care of yourself if you don't know yourself, so spend time with your thoughts and feelings. I misunderstood this for too long. I used to judge myself for not knowing sooner, but the truth is our biggest lessons to pass on come from the hardest, darkest struggles we endure. I could never have written this book or had a leg to stand on without betraying myself over and over for thirty years.

We often judge ourselves for our mistakes. I did for years. I carried guilt and depression and lacked self-worth when I looked in the mirror at what I had chosen for myself. Yes, I said, *chose*. I recognize I chose to betray myself, and only in that realization and acceptance was I able to overcome it. And I never chose over myself again.

There are countless examples of self-betrayal in my life and several stand-out moments where I see how patterns from childhood played out in adulthood. I recognize and have grace for every single human and their experience. Even the worst of us, those that have made our lives feel almost not worth living, are humans experiencing their own journey.

As I recall events in my life that shaped a huge part of my personal development, I want to say that I understand we all do the best we can with what we are given. It isn't always pretty. Some of it is downright embarrassing. But we are always strong enough to decide to be different, anytime.

Several women have contributed their own stories and recollection of events, validating my story has already had a chain reaction for positive change in others.

I am thankful for every single thing that has happened in my life, good and bad. My strength is not a product of these events, but instead, opportunities for my inherent, already present strength to be used. I was given events to be who I have always been. This is a huge takeaway for anyone reading this that has survived something horrific. You are not strong because of what you went through; you already were a warrior. You just needed the battle to prove to yourself you absolutely have what it takes to overcome even the worst situation.

I am a survivor, not a victim. If you identify as a survivor, too, thank yourself for being you. We are never really stuck. We are never really trapped. We may feel that way, but the reality is the more trapped you feel, the deeper you have to dig into your warrior archetype to overcome. She's there, she's always been there.

Although my story does not involve sexual assault, the #metoo movement showed the power of women telling their stories. It took one story, then another, then another. My hope is that this book gives you permission to speak freely your truth, as I am mine. Silence enables abuse and it causes more pain. My voice and yours will heal others, even if we never meet. These moments aren't about being fearless but being brave. Bravery is doing something that does give you fear and doing it anyway. You don't need my permission, but if it helps, then here it is.

My path has always spelled out strength or weakness in some way. I was an athlete and a competitive bodybuilder, requiring me to be strong as a physical specimen. Being a doctor required me to be strong for my patients. And leaving an abusive relationship? Wow, seismic strength.

In my work, I do a lot with physical fitness or weight loss medicine that takes a lot of mental strength. Fitness is not the current focus necessarily, but I was such a disciplined person. I thought I was mentally strong before this relationship. Things were happening, but that was before I lost my whole world. I thought I was strong, then I went through this decade-long juggernaut, and my checkpoints of strength fell down one by one. I'm not sure what makes me more qualified to talk about self-care—my personal life or my professional credentials. In reality, the combination represents my one real life. I believe you will learn a lot from it.

I work full-time telemedicine currently but have excelled in many different environments in my professional career, from private practice-based care, to hospitalist, urgent care work, and now, telemedicine thanks to the pandemic and a desire to deliver quality care in a way that represents the future of medicine. Via telemedicine, I spend much more time with my patients and can hold space for their real problems that are the foundation of their medical ones. In a way, my foundation was missing in my own personal life, which may be why I care so much to hear out my patients more than traditional care has allowed.

Even though I do primary care, nine times out of ten, patients have something in their personal life that is making their health secondary. For example, a patient yesterday called me with her husband leaving out of the blue, and I've been working with her for weight loss. It's much more than lab work. I find the mental health side of things and having people actually get to talk about things they're going through makes all the difference in if they get better physically.

Do people naturally open up? They tend to in the second or third visit once they are more comfortable, knowing that I won't just tell them to "eat healthy." I've heard the same tired words! I'm a doctor. I'm a person first and foremost.

Our engagement turns out to be a personal relationship. Patients confide in me. We're trying to resolve why they are not practicing self-care, not just that they want to look like the beautiful rose, but also, how to nurture the strength of their beauty and the beauty of their strength.

I think of two young girls that were sisters, sixteen and nineteen years old, and when I was their doctor, we found out that their stepfather had been molesting them for years. Watching these girls go through the mental transformation over a year was intense. I remember feeling ill-equipped, but I also recognized I was one of the first people who knew this information and could provide some help, any help. The gravity of my position as someone people trusted started to hit home, while I was hiding my own private life disaster. Everyone has a battle the public doesn't see, and I approach every visit with this in mind.

No matter what patients come in for, there is always something else underlining the symptoms or condition. That's how I feel with my story. It happened to me. I do all this health and fitness and made it look really easy for a long time, then at some point, I completely lost my drive. I lost everything. Now that I've been through that, I look at patients differently. We're not just handling weight loss. Patients have opened up to me about abusive relationships, but it takes time. They're scared I am going to run to the police even though they know it's confidential. Everything resembles fear in that type of relationship, and I know what that feels like.

I was the image of fitness, yet behind closed doors, my days were full of stress, anxiety, and trying to ward off the next blows of abuse. Earlier photos of me are the epitome of strength and then this one relationship tore my world apart. It was a massacre.

I didn't have an emphasis on self-love, identity, and confidence. I relied on outside factors such as relationships, technology, and image.

Discord and disconnect affects the body. Change the clothes, change the profession. Doctors are no different.

I was an athlete my whole life, starting early on, and then I played club sports in college. In med school, I worked out a lot for obvious signs of stress and feeling overextended. When I found a team of coaches that did this bodybuilding thing, I recruited my dear friend, Karla, to join me. She was a police officer in the military (and is currently in the FBI), so surely, she could handle the rigor and tenacity of building herself up, alongside me, and we could cheer each other on. We were strong in sticking with very restrictive diets and working out several hours a day, while keeping up our career trajectory. Our self-esteem was intact. Or so, I thought. We were both drowning in abusive relationships.

The goal of sharing my story is to give permission to other women and men who have been through or are going through similar situations and are looking for their own strength. I am writing this with the intention of telling my dark truth to shed a light for others, because the statistics are far too concerning to stay silent. I see the world, my life, and everyone involved as a product of our own environment and how we choose to respond to adversity. I have grace for every single human, despite how sadistic actions were. We are all humans trying to survive this world, and survival is ugly. None of us want to dwell on things we did during survival. Our ego would much rather paint a picture of triumph and perfection, but no one has a life as such. Revenge doesn't make anyone feel any better, we only feel worse. What I could do with my story is share it and use my voice for others since silence almost killed me. I have learned that sharing your story, your truth, is a powerful self-care practice and one that establishes the path for a fulfilling life journey.

CHAPTER 1
Explosion of Love and Loss

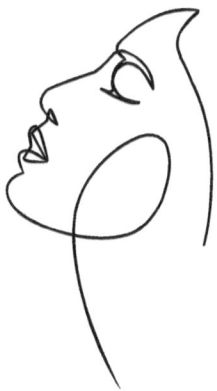

"Romance is the glamour which turns the dust
of everyday life into a golden haze."

—Carolyn Gold Heilbrun

Self-Care RX

PAUL AND I met in the first week of med school. Everyone shouted, "He's not a great guy, stay away!" I met him in a stressful environment so I would blame his behaviors on the stress of us being in school. On paper, he was everything that I would have written down about what I had wanted in a guy. Good-looking, went to the gym, Italian like my family. He bought me gifts, took me on weekend trips.

I think other people saw the warning signs but it's important to acknowledge that we only know what we see. And when we see someone treat us well, but hear otherwise, it's hard to convince our eyes what our ears are told unless we see it ourselves. This was a big lesson for me. I felt a really strong connection to him, and as another story tells later, that electric connection I felt was actually my intuition giving off warning signs. It felt exciting in my twenty-two-year-old heart! However, if I were to recognize this same feeling today, it would be telling me to run the other way, that this was dangerous. I was emotionally ill-equipped to recognize good signs from bad. Emotional maturity is a game changer.

I met the family pretty soon. Pay close attention to the parents. Heed the warning signs. Everything really does stem from our family upbringing. I have a lot more insight into this these days from my own journey. I remember watching how he'd treat his mother, adoring her and praising her at all costs. I also saw him scream at her and kick her out of our home. I felt bad for her because her son was her prize, yet he would turn on her the second he was challenged. We had our share of arguments, but I felt very stuck in the middle of another family's chaos in which I would eventually become the subject of blame. This would play out in the end of the relationship pretty extremely.

Also, after they'd put me down, when I would fight back or start speaking up against it, I was blamed as the problem. I was "rude," "the competitive one." I didn't realize it then, but I was being set up. I have to say, I have fluency in and compassion for family dynamics like this. I think we all do the best we can, but the whole tornado of chaos strengthened until the end. When you start standing up for yourself, things get worse. This is a part of the process of choosing to stay silent in the face of bad behavior, and the fight sometimes isn't worth it.

At first, the family was wonderful. First, they accepted me into this big Italian family as my second family. Come to find out, years later, the mother seemed to have the same issues. Three or four years after we got engaged, I started seeing the light switch between the family members go off. Then I started seeing the same scenarios. She wanted to be my best friend, would buy me gifts and take me to spa days, a shopping day, get to know me, and she wanted to know all of my life story. She seemed like a really nice person, then this competitive behavior ensued. She put me down all the time, my job, my family, and darling son, Paul, followed her the same way. I thought I had this great relationship and then as soon as it got more serious, I saw all the negative signs. His parents did not live near us, so I didn't have to deal with it all the time.

My confidence was at an all-time high at twenty-two years old. I was very focused. I didn't struggle with undergrad, but things seemed easier in med school. The amount of information was difficult, but everything made sense. In undergrad, you're forced to swallow the medicine of taking classes you're not interested in like everyone else. I was doing great. My grades were better than ever. I worked out like crazy. I was a pretty well-rounded individual with this boyfriend who treated me like gold. I thought I was the luckiest person ever.

Three years into school, we were figuring out where we wanted to do residency together. It's complicated to get into the same place with another person. We had to be sure of how serious we were because this would require moving and staying in the same place for three to five years in the same program. It was a big life decision. There were definitely warning signs during this time.

My engagement was very extravagant. Being younger, twenty-five at the time, I thought it was amazing. He flew me on a surprise trip to Napa for a week and proposed to me there. He was hiding a lot. I don't think anybody saw how bad it would eventually become. I was young and liked that arrogant, young guy, never suspecting he was dangerous. Nobody had anything criminal on him or anything.

We ended up matching together at the same program. I think that is where the beginning of the end started. We were both in different fields at the same hospital. He was in surgery. The environment I was in versus the environment he was in was very different. General practitioners are pretty empathic and like to heal everybody and get to know people, whereas the older physicians, "attendings," were all about the cars, money, and dating girls half their age. These elder gents encouraged that behavior for him even though he was engaged. I also don't think anyone realized early on that he was mentally unstable. He liked that world. They would take him on trips to Europe, buy him expensive things and entice him into strip clubs. This kind of behavior was the norm amongst some physicians connected to my fiancé while my work environment fostered the betterment of society.

I protested Paul's behavior when I witnessed it, but I honestly didn't realize how much of it was going on. When you're working eighty-hour work weeks and don't suspect anything, it's easy for someone to create an entirely different life and image without your knowledge. This was a downside in being in a relationship with someone in equal professions, and one person seizing this opportunity.

The physical abuse started, but if I would try to call him out on it or threaten to leave, he would lose control. What I also didn't realize is he would lie excessively. *We had a boat. We were going on exclusive trips around the world.* I look back and remember him telling me things that were not true. *His family had a house in Italy.* He was a habitual liar and very convincing. I never knew what he was telling people at work because I didn't see him during the day. He tried to create a larger-than-life image that portrayed a lifestyle way beyond our means to match that of the seasoned surgeons twice his age. His childhood was one of privilege, however. He went to private schools at $50,000 a year. He had a fairly easy life growing up, which bred entitlement in my opinion.

Homeschooled in Victimization

My own father grew up poor alongside his brother. His parents got divorced at the age of five and he didn't come from much thereafter but made life work. My dad was driven to go to medical school, being the first one to go to college even. His father worked for the NYPD. Italian family. Discipline was physical. That was normal for them. Physical violence was discipline. It was never called "abuse." I grew up thinking that, too. I did something wrong; therefore, this is what happened. I didn't realize until I was like fifteen that this didn't happen in every household. I remember sitting at lunch in high school with the girls' basketball team. We ate together on game days. Somehow the subject came up around the table of how everyone was disciplined in their home. I was the only one who was physically hit for discipline. When I had said this out loud, the whole table stopped eating and looked at me in shock. As if high school isn't vulnerable enough! Needless to say, I had said too much without realizing it. It also created resentment towards my family that not everyone had that experience. In retrospect, I think my father didn't know how to handle a teenage girl. He wanted me to be a star athlete, period.

My parents also separated when I was a sophomore in high school, prime maturation age. I was taking AP classes, playing three varsity sports, and had little to no emotional maturity. Just a lot of anger and resentment. Fortunately, I had a solid friend group. Without them, I don't know what I may have gotten into in my teenage depression.

The punishments, like taking away my makeup, had a big effect on my physical appearance and self-esteem. The punishment, although from an adult perspective seemed like taking away luxuries, really affected my psyche and how I viewed myself. I interpreted it as my punishment was to be "ugly" if I did something wrong. I don't think this was intended, but as an adult, I'm hyper-aware of how things that seem little are a big world to a teenage girl. In contrast, sorority life felt like a whole new world.

To this day, my father would stand by his behavior that it was never an abusive situation. They say a bit of delusion is cultivated when you come from nothing. First, college, then medical school and not only, but to be a cardiologist. He made so much of himself from nothing.

Dad thought if I could make me be a tom boy and avoid boys, boys wouldn't like me. He thought, I want her to be a *strong, badass kind of girl*. This was my earlier condition for "strength." He would say things like, "My daughter will never be a cheerleader." It was not an option. That was equated with pretty, prissy girls in his mind. I was put in soccer and basketball. When I would get in trouble, he would take my hairdryer and brush away.

All this for years has to do with how you view yourself when you become a woman. When I went to college, I had no idea how to apply my makeup. I joined a sorority where these girls were bona fide dolls all the time. I didn't know how to be this way. They accepted me. I went to rush, and it was a grand production. I didn't know anyone where I went to college. It was my way of meeting new people. I just went for it. I remember wearing jean shorts, a tank top and sneakers to rush. All of these girls were in cute sundresses and wedges with hair and makeup totally packaged up.

What class did I miss that taught you how to make yourself up this way? I was struggling how I was as an individual. I wasn't allowed to be that way. Then when I went that route, I loved femininity and embraced it. It wasn't what my dad made it out to be. I could be feminine and not weak. I had boyfriends in college, but when I met Paul in med school, I had come out of college and started to figure out who I was and how I wanted to look.

I guess you could say Paul reinforced my new appearance, and I could never know that he was a narcissist. Part of the narcissistic relationship is in the beginning, *love bombing*, displaying so much affection and showering you with attention. The feeling is like hearts floating in an emoji. They tell you that you're the greatest thing since sliced bread. This phase lasted perhaps a year and a half. The negative comments did not start until after this. I met this guy who would buy me dresses and show me off. I had never had somebody treat me like that before. He made me feel sexy after being raised with the notion that sexiness, or heightened sex appeal, was a bad thing. It actually felt awesome. I think the combination of my struggle with how to be feminine, and his personality disorder, the nature of that and how he got girls into a relationship with him, morphed into a perfect mold. He made me feel amazing, like I was the world. I felt like that was L-O-V-E and this was it. I was in 100 percent.

Psych Central sums up what I was in for: "The intensity of

being married to a narcissist is similar to a having another full-time job as the narcissist tends to dump on their spouse anything they don't want to handle. Frequently, the spouse neglects themselves for the sake of the narcissist by justifying that the reduced anger is worth the extra effort. Unfortunately, life doesn't work this way as most spouses only wind up exhausted in the end."

Think about that. How do you feel? I get the sense of entrapment even writing it.

Who is the person behind this complex medical health condition? Definitely not who I thought loved me. They simply do not *love*. Narcissists are incapable of loving others. They have low empathy, a grandiose or inflated sense of self, and an extreme need for admiration and attention.

All Threats Are Serious

There was a handful of times when we were in med school that things became physical. Compared to the years we were together and all of the good things he had done, I forgave.

One time, I needed a book to study with and we had one copy. We shared books. Why buy two copies if we lived together? He said, "It's mine."

I said playfully, "You're not using it." He was so stuck on the fact that it wasn't my book since it had his name on the inside. I went over and said, "I'm going to take it. I need this and it's ridiculous that you wouldn't let me use it." And *BAM!* He completely close-lined me to the floor.

Someone witnessed that because we had a friend staying with us for a few months. He ended up leaving over this incident because he just couldn't believe that had happened. He tried to help me up and told Paul to get the hell away from me. We got in the car and left. Meantime, my ex sat down to go back to studying and acted like nothing had happened. This was pretty normal. His ability to calmly study for hours after an incident was chilling. He was never shaken by his actions, whereas I would be hysterical and heartbroken.

Therapist Weatherly Camacho, LPC, calls the consequences of this treatment "death by paper cuts." It's little jabs all the time. When they give you jabs, they might build you up in a couple of days. It's an intentional cycle. It's an organic part of their personality. They feel the need to have someone to completely control. Depending on how they feel in that moment, they will do what they need to do to keep you in line. They feel good about themselves when they need it. It's crazy because you don't realize it's happening. Camacho specializes in narcissistic abuse.

Tearing something down only makes room to build something new. Rock bottom isn't the end to something old but the start of a new life with a clean slate.

For me, rock bottom was an abusive relationship.

Names I was called:

Cunt.

Whore.

Slut.

Ugly.

Fat and used up.

Who do you picture when you think about someone in a verbally or physically abusive relationship? What's the picture in your mind?

The caveat is that I may be the last person you'd expect. I am educated, successful in my work, overall happy, physically strong, independent financially, and I have pretty average self-esteem. How did I get here? Very slowly.

Self-Care RX

If a man were to hit you on the first date, you wouldn't go out with him again. But what if he waits until the fiftieth date? It seems more like an outlier in behavior relative to the rest of the relationship. It's easy to say he "snapped, it was a very bad day," and sympathize that "we all have rock bottom days." The aggressor may have some reason why he snapped, and turn it around to say something like, "I'm just so scared of losing the love of my life." How do you walk away in that one singular moment? You don't. And if you're thinking you'd leave in that moment because of one bad day, I hate to tell you that you're probably wrong.

I went into medicine to help people, so why would I turn my back on the person I love because of one bad day? We always hear that couples fight behind closed doors. We don't really know what "normal" is for anyone else.

This is not to excuse staying with someone that harms you, but to explain the line of thinking that occurs in the early stages of an evolving abusive relationship from my point of view—and to acknowledge that it's not logical. The aggressor makes you believe you can help them, and that their actions are because they love you. This clearly does not make logical sense, again, but it's a slow mind game they start to play with you. The first time this happens, the tone has been set for the next time…because there will be a next time. And you don't see it coming.

I once asked a friend amidst leaving an abusive relationship if he had ever hit her. She said, "No, he smashed my television, but he's never hit me. I don't think he'd do that!" My response was it will only be a matter of time. These things escalate over time. The cycle may be slow or rapid. Her ex ended up threatening to harm her family and almost killed her dog. Retrospect is everything. Knowing what I know now, any sign of violence—even toward an object—is a sign of potential escalation and danger.

You start to feel that if you pay more attention to them, cater to them, even in little ways, that you may prevent another "rock bottom" day like the one I've mentioned. They get more attention. Time goes by, and they do show you appreciation, shower you with love in many ways for weeks, months, maybe a year.

Then the second time occurs. Be careful when your inner chatter overtakes common sense because your actions start to follow the beliefs in your head. Here is an example:

How could this happen again? I was doing everything to help him. He had another bad day. He feigned tears about being fearful of me leaving because I had been so good to him. He really felt like I didn't love him? How could this be true since I'd shown him 1,000 ways, even doing laundry, cooking dinner, giving him space, letting him have his hobbies and be himself? He must be under a lot of stress, clearly this is another really bad day. We have a life together; we can fix this! True love conquers all, right? Couples make it through the worst time.

I told myself a million lies and believed them. We were both smart people. So smart we were on our way to becoming respected doctors. Surely, we could figure this out. *He's not some degenerate—this must be an extreme stress reaction.*

Then the third instance occurred.

The time I realized things were not normal was one night in our apartment. I don't remember what the argument was about, but it wasn't something important. …Just another "bad day." The fight escalated into intense screaming and insults. I wasn't backing down whatever the topic was. I knew that whatever names he called me were uncalled for and I held him to it. When he started to lose the verbal fight, he didn't "hit" me; he grabbed my body and slammed me onto the ground. This is not something you see coming when it's your partner. He kicked me and kept hitting me on the ground. I froze. Keep in mind I'm a black belt in Tae Kwon

Do and a competitive athlete, with a strong personality. You'd think *kick his ass*, right? I felt completely emotionally broken. Frozen. The physical part hurt, but honestly, I didn't feel physical pain; I felt emotional pain and numb. I just felt like I had lost. I felt helplessness.

I laid there crying for a while. He went back to his desk and continued to study. Only a psychopath could beat up his girlfriend, then calmly go back to studying without a flinch.

I took a bath, closed the door and decided to simply remove myself for a minute, reset. *What the hell just happened?* It's so fast you can't even comprehend it when it happens to you versus when you are watching someone else.

Somehow the fight restarted verbally, while I was in the bathtub trying to decompress. I was crying and yelling back, so angry and defeated. How does he not look at me and feel the slightest bit sorry? The next thing I knew, he came into the bathroom, grabbed the back of my neck, and pushed my head down into the bathtub water face first. It was maybe five seconds in reality, but the experience felt like infinity. Go ahead and count five seconds, even three. Was he trying to kill me? No, but scare me into submission? Yes. Then he went back to studying calmly.

I knew that this was not sustainable, not something I wanted. Still in disbelief, I went to work the next day trying to hold it together the best I could, but only able to focus on what happened the previous night. Both of us excelled in the workplace and were masters of compartmentalization. The fact that I was able to go to work and perform the next day I believe was a result of my rigorous athletic training. It isn't a bad skill to have, but I used this skill in the extreme to my own detriment. In athletics, you leave everything going on in your life off the court and focus on the game. I was stellar at this. It's why I was able to excel in medical school and the long hours of training, with an eye on the prize. I can rest when it's over. Note: This skill shouldn't have been needed in a relationship. I emphasize this point because so many of us possess it, whether it be extreme focus or determination, ambition, but it should not be triggered or accessed in the manner I am speaking of in a romantic relationship. Love does not demand this of you.

Three months later, we became engaged.

The ability to act in that way and immediately go back to whatever he was doing was the norm for him. He would go to work, act like nothing happened. It was amazing. Every time it happened, over and over in my head, I would say, *this is wrong. I don't deserve this.* I never thought it was okay and there was never a good excuse.

My self-esteem plummeted because I kept going back, knowing it was wrong. I could not tell anybody because if you tell your friends, they will never forgive your partner, and you're usually held accountable by them to do something about it. I knew as soon as I said it out loud, it had to be over. If I tried to fix it, people would think I was crazy. It was not "often," and I kept telling myself he was under a lot of stress. Then I started getting to the place that I thought he needed help and that I was the only person to understand this. I started justifying his behavior. And maybe to help myself feel better. Looking back, it doesn't even feel like me. He wouldn't necessarily say I'm sorry, but he would do something after us not speaking for a couple of days; he would book a weekend getaway to "start fresh and clear our heads." I thought, *we can get past this.*

We didn't get past it. These abusive episodes happened nine or ten times in eight years. It got worse later because he started breaking down. The more I started catching on to his lies and realizing he was not who he said he was, the angrier he became. He didn't know how to react to somebody telling him he was basically a fraud. There were times he would try to strangle me, not to kill me, but to scare me or make me submit. It was pure reaction, no thought. If I had marks, his behavior would have to be explained. If he grabbed my neck or threw me on the ground, something that wouldn't necessarily leave a bruise like a black eye, he wouldn't be held accountable. To this day, I don't know if this was intentional, but I don't recall having visible marks.

The guy who had witnessed the book incident had been our mutual friend. My ex gets people to be infatuated with him whether from a friendship standpoint or romantic standpoint. It happened at work and I still see it in how people talk about him: "He's such a great guy. He's so ambitious." He would extend a "helping hand" to people and come across like he really cares about your aspirations such as starting a business. This mutual friend was living with us after Paul singularly invited him to live with us, rent-free, because he was trying to get started on his own career. He would do anything, incredible things, to get someone to like him. That distorted support system only reinforced his abusive behavior.

CHAPTER 2
Too Smart, Rich or Famous to be Sick

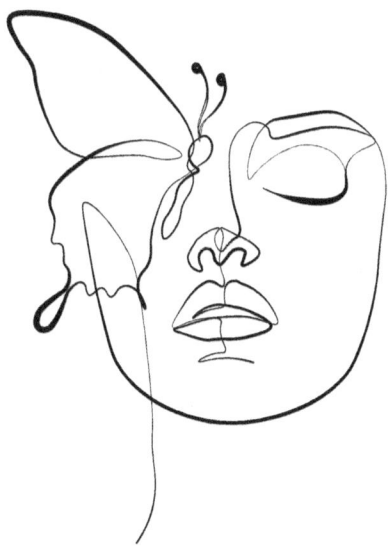

"Illusion is the first of all pleasures."

—Voltaire

We had bought a house in the suburbs where people mow their grass on Sundays. This type of neighborhood mirroring my childhood and sense of family was what I wanted at the time. I thought, *we're starting our life together*! It went the completely opposite direction. He took the mortgage out and I wanted both of our names on the house, which he agreed to. We went house hunting, and we were standing in our house together with him asking if this is the one. Exactly what you picture on HGTV!

As soon as he signed and we moved in, Paul spoke to me like a roommate or servant. "Don't dirty my house." "I can kick you out anytime." As soon as he had something on paper to hold over me, the notion of "our future" was a big façade. He couldn't afford the house on his own though. He could make you feel like you were everything at the moment he needed you to be for his sole gain.

What about school during all of this chaos? I would have people cover for me here and there, but I never took a leave. I told my boss at some point, when things were really bad because it was showing in my work. People knew something was wrong. No one asked me, but I don't think I would have been honest if they had. I wasn't ready to come to terms yet.

Seven years in, the last year, was the worst. It was almost like Paul performed better at work when something was wrong at home. People praised him left and right. He was very much about the letters along his name, his title, his resume. He would talk about his credentials as soon as he met someone and probably tell you he had a Porsche. He started becoming that way in residency. Once people realized something was going on, what happened was

I became extremely isolated. I had a couple of people stand by me, but all these mutual friends, which were the bulk since we had moved there together, kind of stood back and dispersed. No one wanted to get involved. This was the result of my resilience and silence. In no one knowing what to believe, it gave him a platform to say whatever he wanted first, while I continued to keep my private life private.

When the serious issues started coming to light, people did not want to be a part of it at all. At one point, Paul disappeared, just didn't come home for a couple of days. His parents had bought a vacation home about ten minutes away. I thought he was staying there. He was avoiding me out of the blue.

It was the one-year anniversary of another resident's suicide. My ex was the last person to see him alive. This person was the all-star resident. Everyone loved him. He always had a smile on his face and had fellowships lined up for him. He invited people out one night a month before he was set to graduate. My ex stayed out with him for a while then they parted ways. My ex woke up the next morning and heard about his death. He had called people before leaving the house. That is the story I got from everybody. Paul was the last person to see him, so he felt a lot of guilt over the guy not telling him specifically what was going on. He wasn't someone you would have suspected struggling based on his happy demeanor at work. This tragedy definitely catapulted Paul's behavior. I mistook it as new behavior, but it was escalation of old behavior under extreme stress. He hit a breaking point.

When Paul started doing crazy things, like planning trips to Europe, I thought, okay, he needs to get away. I was manufacturing reasons. I didn't know how much partying he was doing when he was away. I finally found out he was taking girls to his parents' house.

I was on call with a girl he was sleeping with, and she was

a medical student. We were on call the same night I found out. Feeling the rage inside, before confronting her, I thought, is this worth losing my job over? I went to bad places in my head. It was a Sunday, and I was coming in that night. We weren't talking. We didn't break up. We were just having an issue. As I was heading into work, this girl walked out, which was weird because her class had graduated the day before. Why was she in the hospital? Two minutes later, I got a call from one of my good friends in the residency program. Apparently, she had walked in on them in the call room. They were eating dinner together, but it was understood what was happening.

I did confront her. She denied it. I continued: "Do you realize we have been together for seven years? We're engaged. I still have my ring on." She said they were just hanging out. You get to know all the medical students. Everyone knows everyone. She knew we were together.

I threw up a few times at work from the devastation. My good friends and co-residents checked on me and luckily, one girl I knew was also on call and stayed with me all night, while another girl covered admissions for me. Another friend made me dinner. One of the amazing parts of residency is you form a family. You watch out for each other. These people may have saved my life in ways to come and kept me from making bad decisions out of anger that may have affected my career. Complete survival mode was engaged, and it's ugly.

Making friends had never been an issue for me, and just like childhood, I don't know what I would have done without them around. When your whole world is flipped upside down and you have to show up to work, in the same building with people hurting you, you start to lose sight of reality and question if revenge is worth losing your job over. I had actually sent the medical student a message on Facebook a few days later our of extreme anger, which I was reprimanded for. But the humanity of my boss understood I was going through hell and told me to take some time. I was surrounded by great people, even though it took me the absolute extreme to speak up.

Paul avoided me for days. One night, he came home to get clothes and said, "We're not talking. I'm just here to get clothes." He refused to talk. Then he eventually got cavalier about it: "Yeah, I like sleeping with eighteen-year-old girls," and started saying horrible things after I pressed him. "They give me what I want." Apparently, he was sleeping with people all over town. He bragged that he wouldn't even know the girls' names if he saw them on the street, that he wouldn't even recognize them, he had so many.

Paul looked like an absolute monster at that point. We didn't have a fight for all this to be instigated. People asked me if he was doing drugs.

After weeks of realizing my whole engagement was over, I had decided to move out. I found a place and was starting to move on. He came back in the middle of the night and told me if I didn't give him another chance, he would commit suicide.

Directory of Mania

Several weeks later, I let him back in. What do they say about witches and vampires? You have to invite them in! He went to a therapist and took me with him. They diagnosed him with bi-polar disorder. He tried to blame this on a manic episode. People with true mania do things like go sleep with people, take trips. He had gone skydiving twice in one day. People typically break in their late twenties or early thirties.

Once we had a diagnosis, I felt guilty instantly for leaving him. I wanted to, but I felt like I was deserting someone. I somehow convinced myself that this was all because of a treatable mental illness, and he wanted my help recovering. As a doctor, I fully understood what this meant. It also created more of a story for me to convince myself to try again. This pulled on my doctor strings and empathy.

His parents would just take him out to another dinner because of his public image. They never quite got it. I went to therapy with him a handful of times, and it felt like he was trying to convince me how sorry he was rather than it being therapy for him. It was a big show looking back. He knew he would now lose me with good reason and resorted to a mindset of *I'll do everything to keep you.* He was given prescription medication. He took it for a month or two. Then he simply lied about taking it.

Within that time, we had actually decided to try to plan a wedding. I know…it's terrible, embarrassing to even say it right now. He wanted to go cake tasting and look at venues. At this point, we had been "engaged" for four or five years. We started this whole charade, setting a date and place. All of my friends remind me that I never talked about my wedding or got excited about planning it. It's because I was embarrassed for taking him back. The cheating became so public. He was open about everything to everybody, bragging about the trips and girls, bringing them out with our mutual friends. It went from us looking like this couple that had it together and having issues at home, to him just throwing it all over the place and vomiting all of his indiscretions. It was a very embarrassing time for me. I had just gotten promoted to chief resident. As soon as work was getting really good and affirming my achievements, culminating my efforts for many years, the personal life went to hell.

Have you ever watched "Big Little Lies?" Nicole Kidman's storyline is so close to my situation. Watching her husband be so "perfect" (even down to how sterile and organized their house was) and overly affectionate at times and then the rage that overtakes him (mostly the scene when the toys are on the floor) gave me chills because that is exactly the type of abusive relationship I was in (minus the rape). She was a lawyer, so most people would say she should "know better" but she didn't. And he lost control and almost killed her when she tried to leave and found out, which is what happened to me also. Leaving is scary because deep down, you know the abuser is capable of anything.

There's also a lot of talk in the sports world about domestic violence lately. Ohio State University head coach, Urban Meyer, was suspended for potentially knowing about his assistant coach being violent at home towards his wife and not doing anything about it or reporting it. The wife had gotten a restraining order, which is what made it public, and the wife said she told others back in 2015 about the abuse and everyone overlooked it. I wonder if this was for the sake of football, or maybe the idea of "it's not affecting our work here" played a role.

Are the same repercussions happening in jobs not in the public eye? Lots of people knew about my ex, but it was overlooked as gossip, I was being dramatic, or that he's functioning fine at work so what happens at home isn't our business. Just made me think do these things happen to celebrities to make a point but not to those where it can be easily ignored. No one wants to step up against a coworker or worse, a friend or family member that they may *know* is abusive. Why this is I'm not sure I can fully answer—forget chivalry; this is enabling. It's like that scenario where you have to tell your girlfriend her husband is cheating. Will she believe you? Will she leave? What about looking at a friend and saying, "I know you're hitting your wife and I'm going to the police or your boss?" This might even be a dangerous situation, depending how volatile the person is.

It's a tricky situation, but so relevant right now in the news.

Urban Meyer wasn't the abusive one; he just knew and did nothing and therefore, got suspended.

I'm not sure there is a playbook for how to approach a friend suspected of abuse. However, I do know that silence among friends feels like abandonment. We always ask why people don't do something when they see a wrong; it's a never-ending question. We won't ever know the answer. I always felt so angry for those that knew what was happening and continued to enable him. There's a part in the movie "Enough" starring Jennifer Lopez when she shows her mother-in-law a facial bruise her husband gave her. The mother-in-law's response is, "What did you do?" Others' silence felt like this internally.

The following statistics released by Centers for Disease Control (CDC) and RAINN leave a feeling of shock and helplessness from the numbers alone, but if we think of every number as a life impacted, we think of a bottomless pit of destroyed lives, lost potential, and damaged psyches.

Survivors—particularly women due to other complexities and pressures in their identity—must know that they are not alone in their experiences. They must know that they can do their part in stopping a destructive cycle. I'm a millennial doctor. I experienced this firsthand.

- On average, 24 people per minute are victims of rape, physical violence or stalking by an intimate partner in the United States—more than 12 million women and men over the course of a year.
- Nearly 3 in 10 women (29%) and 1 in 10 men (10%) in the US have experienced rape, physical violence and/or stalking by a partner and report a related impact on their mental functioning.

- Nearly, 15% of women (14.8%) and 4% of men have been injured as a result of intimate partner violence (IPV) that included rape, physical violence and/or stalking by an intimate partner in their lifetime.
- 1 in 4 women (24.3%) and 1 in 7 men (13.8%) aged 18 and older in the United States have been the victim of severe physical violence by an intimate partner in their lifetime.
- IPV alone affects more than 12 million people each year.
- More than 1 in 3 women (35.6%) and more than 1 in 4 men (28.5%) in the United States have experienced rape, physical violence and/or stalking by an intimate partner in their lifetime.
- Nearly half of all women and men in the United States have experienced psychological aggression by an intimate partner in their lifetime (48.4% and 48.8%, respectively).
- Females ages 18 to 24 and 25 to 34 generally experienced the highest rates of intimate partner violence.
- From 1994 to 2010, about 4 in 5 victims of intimate partner violence were female.
- Most female victims of intimate partner violence were previously victimized by the same offender, including 77% of females ages 18 to 24, 76% of females ages 25 to 34, and 81% of females ages 35 to 49.

I want you to think about your three best friends. Statistically, one of them will experience some level of domestic violence. Of my core friend group, three of eight have experienced domestic violence; we are in our mid-thirties. Some of those stories are in this book.

CHAPTER 3

Disappearance of Self and Census

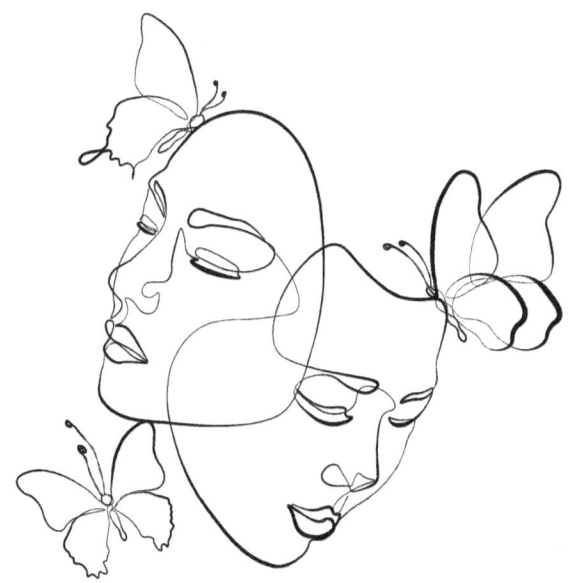

"The value of life can be measured by how many times your soul has been deeply stirred."

—Soichiro Honda

Self-Care RX

There are explicit rules of an unhealthy relationship designed to cause isolation and confusion.

In front of others, Paul would tell me how proud he was and brag about me. Behind closed doors, he always put me down for what I did. There is this thing in medicine; he is considered a specialist and I'm a general doctor. Many people think that specialists are the elite. This mentality showed in his attendings. They all thought they were gods, and could have whatever girls, cars, adventures. In my program, everyone was down to earth and wanted to be doctors. Two different worlds.

After all this, I realized I was a very anxious person, but I didn't recognize why. It was what I went home to. I used to be someone who could handle a lot. It was out of character for me not to be able to handle five or six things at once. I was chief resident when I found out about that girl. One of my best friends had been on call with me. We had just finished signing out patients with the group and the whole group left, and I just lost it. I started crying hysterically. It all came out then. She covered for me a lot. I would dip out or not be present for an hour or two at a time for therapy for him or he was having a crisis, something stressful, then people would say that I got a lot of slack. I had to deal with that while not telling everyone what was happening. That year was harder than it should have been. People didn't understand what was happening with me. I also didn't want to bring my personal life to work.

When I found out he was sleeping with that girl, my boss gave me the day off and covered for me. He let other attendings know there was stuff going on and they reached out. When I ended up taking him back and planning a wedding, it was like I wasn't any better, but the sympathy was gone. They just wanted me to get back to work. My boss at the time was a father figure, wanting everyone to be a good doctor and good at life. If I had any other boss in that hospital, they would not have understood. He was shocked. He knew the people influencing my ex, but he couldn't do anything about it. He set me up with my ex's boss for a one-on-one meeting, informing him some things were going on with Paul. We met, but he was emphasizing, "If something is going on, he'll have to take a leave of absence and put it on job applications and explain why. It's a lot more paperwork than it's worth. How bad is this really?"

It was hard to tell them what was really happening. On the theme of erratic behavior, I explained that he was on a downward spiral and that he was going to have a nervous breakdown. He specifically asked me if I thought he would commit suicide because a year prior, a resident had. I didn't answer yes or no. He had threatened but at that point, had never truly attempted suicide. Then everything hit the destruction button.

This type of personality is so intricate. The way that my therapist has explained *malignant narcissism* is they have no sense of self and they don't know who they are. They will take bits of pieces from things of people around them and then put that person down. They want to be the person but get threatened by their completeness and twist the situation to be negative in order to make themselves feel better. How they are feeling that day dictates if they are going to build the person up or tear them down.

I had a relationship under this umbrella for years. What unexpected things happened to me during the process? How did it change me? With someone like this, and this has happened to others speaking out, is you completely lose who you are. You're not doing anything for yourself anymore. Everything you are doing is to keep that person from causing chaos. If things are stable, narcissists want to throw a wrench into the mix. If you're doing great, they want to screw that up for you. You start altering things in your daily life to tiptoe around what you've learned may set this person off. For example, if there was a single dish on the counter, he might come home and throw that dish on the floor and say, "This is a pig stie. I can't believe you want to live this way." It was always somehow narrated as, "I can't believe you are this disgusting and okay with this level of cleanliness. Something is wrong with you as a person." Not like, "Hey, can we clean the place today?" A more neutral approach!

That goes from appearance to intellect. He would feel threatened and try to make me feel less confident. Over time, especially in eight years, you learn what they are going to go after. Little things that over time, build up. You slowly start changing. Eight years later, I'm basically living to not piss this person off—that was my routine. It had nothing to do with doing anything to make me happy. I was living on an electricity volt of anxiety. It's not bread-and-butter depression or anxiety but rather, psychological complications that are manifestations of C-PTSD (complex post-traumatic stress disorder), which is what I have.

You can't identify a narcissist unless you get to know them. It's a cycle of psychological abuse you can't readily see. This also adds time to the relationship clock. By the time I had asked for help things were so bad. I was terrified to speak to my ex's boss, absolutely terrified. Not because of him, but because how do you say what is really going on in a way that is professional? I had a hard time finding the words. When he asked me if I thought he would commit suicide, I didn't answer. But looking back, I knew the answer was a potential yes, and my brain went on a fast track to all the consequences of either answer. Looking back, my intuition knew it was possible.

I speak a lot about resident suicide. This topic is conflicting for me to discuss because the way this played out would turn into him holding me hostage by threatening suicide rather than a real attempt. As I discuss this topic, I want to be really clear where my head was and the red flags that signaled "real" versus "fake" in my particular situation, without anyone applying them directly to their own, as everyone's situation is different, and this topic is a deadly one if handled wrong.

I have no doubt that this person was deeply in pain and had loads of unresolved issues. The difference is choosing to project that pain onto others instead of choosing to face their own under-developed areas.

My therapist made me realize none of this was my fault. When I first started seeing her, I thought, *I'm just dealing with someone mentally ill and I'm a doctor and I can't even help my significant other*. I went from that to realizing there was nothing I could have done.

After all of this trauma and victim shaming afterwards, there is something that I think victims of any abuse go through. You somehow feel very isolated and alone because you start to realize no one understands your story no matter how much you try to explain what happens. Victims don't come forward for so many reasons and feeling "different" is a big part of it. It does cause a lot of depression and anxiety. (Wherever you are in the world reading my story, I am empathically telling you now, you are not alone.)

Small talk seems to not make much sense anymore, like nothing small matters so why put in the energy when you don't have energy to give. You don't have energy for things that don't give you something positive so you can barely talk about the weather or gossip. You start to view yourself as some sort of anomaly that no one understands. This causes a great deal of grief for people, like the loss of a life, friends, or your identity.

The Myth of Beauty and the Beast

The delusion is that successful, strong women would not get involved with this type of guy. I'm a doctor. My friend, Karla, is military police.

In short, here is her story that she shares here for potential resonance: "My boyfriend ended up staying two more weeks when I told him to get out. I called his dad and told him to come get him. He left a lot of his stuff and I had to bring it to him at some point. That was the last time I saw him. He wrote a few residual emails, but I didn't answer them. How could I let someone push me around like that? It happens. I almost got arrested one time. The cops came to the house and I was fearful of that because I was walking a dog outside. Somebody yelled down from the balcony about putting the dog on a leash. I went home and told him. He ran to the car and grabbed a knife. He then banged on that guy's door and told him to come out. That dude called the cops, and the cops came to my door. He was hiding in the bathroom. I told the cop he left because he told me to lie. Here I am—a cop! I lied because he told me to. Why would I do that? Anyone can be manipulated by what you think is *love*."

As she was experiencing her own nightmare at home, she saw signs of Paul's abuse. When we were out to dinner with friends, he punched my leg under a table once. The table shook with everyone's foods and drinks tumbling. She and others saw his tantrums as public displays. When we moved into our house, he had the audacity to tell Karla, my friend, "Danielle never cleans anything, the floors are a mess, I am the only one who cleans around here." He would say these things whether I was in the room or not.

At our best friend, Elizabeth's wedding, we were her maids of honor. He was a jackass the entire night. He was upset about not being at another event, a trip, and Elizabeth's wedding ended up being on that weekend. He stayed in the room the whole time and then at the reception, he was standing in the corner by himself. He couldn't even pretend to have fun. He verbally embarrassed me in front of all of my friends as revenge. It's as if he was mad if we had to do something that was centered around someone else, like a wedding. So he tried to ruin the night instead.

Paul mentioned that movie, "Limitless," that his life was this and with all moving so fast and blurry, he barely remembered sleeping with other women. But then of course, he accused me of cheating. Karla's boyfriend did the same. "It started with him being upset about not answering a phone call or text in a timely manner. That was big for me. Just blame. Over and over, you start to think you did fuck up. Doubting yourself of what you know better. You know yourself better than anybody. When somebody starts making you think you're in the wrong and you're not, that's a big sign. You start to believe it yourself that you're not good enough or doing what you're supposed to be doing. Suddenly everything you've ever done was not good enough. Then you have to do more! Mostly to please that person, the system you're living in, things you wouldn't normally do. You start changing. And you're changing for the worst, not the better."

Between Karla and my friend, Dawn, who is also a doctor, they had a front row seat to the horror movie my life was becoming. I believe Dawn's characterization of both of us could not be more accurate though today, it is very difficult for me to share since that version of "Danielle" is now a stranger.

"Without sounding weird and caddy, they came off as a couple as standoffish. She was more reserved. He came off as arrogant. He was interesting to talk to! If there was a topic about me, he would dominate that topic. That was a red flag. She would let him take the spotlight. Getting to know them as a couple, together they were odd. The second year, that's when I got to know the real Danielle at a conference in Kansas City and he was not there. We connected then. Before then, we were just good colleagues. She was a different person when she was not around Paul and we became good friends. She's really strong. I don't want to sound like she is this weak woman. That is not my first impression of her. He talked big talk and she let him do it. Later on, she told me she would confront him on certain things he said in front of her friends. She was not a timid, battered woman. I never got that impression. I don't think anyone noticed she was in an abusive relationship. His personality was just very obvious, that he was full of himself. He was a weird and quirky guy, and she was the nice one. But it wasn't like something seemed wrong enough to investigate. We would laugh about times when they would come to parties separately or driving to other events separately. People who are engaged don't do that. Now I can speculate. They weren't in the most loving relationship, but we just brushed them off as busy. We never saw them holding hands or kissing. They didn't act in love or that they were getting married. Not until he messed up a lot and toward the end, he faked some of that stuff. I rarely saw them being affectionate in public. But sometimes I feel that Danielle is not a mushy, gushy girl either. I would refer to things that I laughed at during the time and she finally told me the back story of usually arguing later over that instance. They were buying a house. None of us had that much money, and 99 percent of us were renting. The first impression we had was, they have their shit together. It's awesome. Then I learned that the day they closed on the house, he tried to slap her and choke her in the car, spatting, 'This is my house, not yours.'"

CHAPTER 4

Leaving the Weight of Someone Else's World

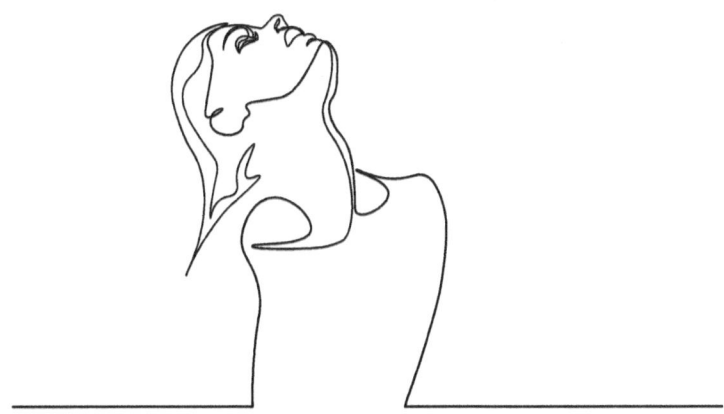

"Life shrinks or expands in proportion to one's courage."

—Anais Nin

Self-Care RX

I HAD JUST PASSED my boards, the last test you have to take for ten whole years! I had signed a contract for a job and was going to take a month off. Paul still had a couple more years of training. Clearly, I was going to start making money and he was not yet. He offered to take me to dinner to celebrate. I got all dressed up on cloud nine.

We were sitting at dinner and talking about my job and the subject of our incomes. I initiated setting up a joint account. We had a wedding date. I always felt like I was doing all the mechanical things you do for a relationship, and it kept getting screwed up. This was May and we were going to marry in September. He became so irate at the fact I said I would give him money, share money, like he needed my help. He took it so horribly wrong that he started yelling at me at the table. We had finished eating. He got up and left. I had been left at plenty of places by him before.

This was the first time I stayed put and finished my wine. I did not care that he left me or if he came back. He never came back. All my friends were out celebrating so I met up with them. He didn't call or text to see if I got home. We always said we didn't want children and then it became an issue later. He had told me that if I got pregnant, it meant abortion. He wanted no part of it. He thought a child would take all of his money and they were simply annoying.

I stayed at my friend's house that night. He didn't call the next day. I stayed there the whole week.

The crazier part was my bachelorette party the following weekend. I went with ten friends. Everybody sensed something was up. We were in Las Vegas. On the last day, at a pool party at Encore Beach Club, we had gotten a table and I looked at all of them and said, "Guys, I'm not getting married. I can't do this." They all started clapping and were fully supportive. They did not want me to marry this man.

I also found out that he had been texting awful things to several of the girls throughout the weekend, trying to ruin our time together. He had been texting me as well, but at some point, I ignored the messages and stayed present with my friends. Here I was at my "bachelorette party," for all he knew still, and he was attempting to ruin every second. I knew I couldn't hide when I was surrounded by the love of my best friends. I had been hiding so much for so long. I also learned they all knew it was bad, even if they didn't know every detail. Your support system can literally save your life.

This example is one of the first real times I silenced my phone in the face of verbal harassment. The significance here for me is I felt physically safe doing so, as I was in another state surrounded by friends. I didn't have to deal with it that night, or the next, just when I eventually went home. I got the sense of what it was like not betraying myself in those few days. It was incredibly liberating, I felt so much myself. I was about to graduate, and I wasn't reliant on anyone nor had I ever been. But I had this overwhelming sense of being okay even if the changes in my life sucked for a while. I was mentally calculating if I had the strength to leave while I was at my bachelorette weekend.

As further significance, I stopped responding to those texts. The danger eventually escalated. Deep down you know it might, but you don't ever really think you're going to be in a dangerous situation until it happens. My friends literally saved my life that weekend just by being present and showing me love.

Getting left at that restaurant was the last straw. I never went home after that besides for moving out. He found me in the hall a couple days after at work and asked if I was leaving him. I replied, with as much strength as I could muster, "Yes, I am leaving you."

He didn't say anything and walked in the other direction. A couple of days later, he didn't show up to work, and everybody was calling his phone. They were worried because of the other resident committing suicide two years prior. Paul didn't answer the calls.

Then someone called me at 2:00 in the afternoon asking if I knew where he was. Paul not showing up to work, at last, due to his own implosion, was like the emperor without clothes on.

I went to the house and it was quiet. I went upstairs and spotted him on the bed with a gun in his hand. He had written suicide notes to his brother and me. I read the note. "I'm sorry I wasn't enough for you, and I'm sorry I hurt you. I don't deserve to be alive." What a pity party on paper! I didn't feel anything. The years had finally caught up to me. I was all out of cares to have for him. I looked at him as I would just another vulnerable human being, not someone I had shared my life and most intimate moments with for eight years. "What are you doing? Snap out of this."

I took the gun away. He stayed in the bed. I placed it on the ledge by the staircase. Things had gotten so horrible, it felt surreal. I talked to him and he was not answering me. I think the real feeling I had here was not taking responsibility for what he said in those notes or what he was doing. Somehow my gut instinct was trying to decide how real this was. And this is going to come across to some as horrible, but with a pattern of this behavior, I don't think I knew what was real anymore. You would think, why didn't she call 9-1-1! Something in me knew if I took my attention off of him all hell would break loose. I felt hostage by the entire situation. Looking back, I should have called 9-1-1, as should anyone in this situation. But in that moment, I feared, if I pick up my phone and give him a second to himself, will he kill himself? Or me? Or run in fear of his job? There's no playbook for this scenario, especially when you don't know what's real.

He looked at me robotically and said, "Are you really leaving me?" Oh boy. Do I say no or yes, and if I say no, I have to eventually tell him that I'm leaving him later? I said, "Yes." He got up calmly and then darted to the staircase to grab the gun. I became hysterical. I thought telling him the truth in that moment was a mistake, that I was making him kill himself. He put the gun in his mouth, crying. Then he said, "I don't know what is better. Killing myself and making you live with it for the rest of your life or taking you with me."

He eventually took the gun away from his mouth and was holding it. He shut his eyes for a second. I tackled him and kicked the gun away from him. I didn't know how to handle a gun or if it was loaded. I had no idea!

I got the gun and took it downstairs. At one point, I was holding him on the floor. I didn't stand a chance physically except that he was so emotionally wrecked. Then he fumbled with pills. When he put the pills in his mouth, he didn't actually swallow them that I could see. It was like a kid missing his mouth but pretending to shove them all back and missing. This was extreme, but looking back, he wasn't trying to harm himself. My doctor brain was on fire; he wasn't drowsy, yet he should have been if he took them. I also didn't know if he took any prior.

Not calling 9-1-1 is one of my biggest regrets. But I'm here to be honest about the pressures you have in a career in medicine. Mental health is not something we can have on our record; there are potential repercussions. This is how deep this rabbit hole went in my past life, of protecting myself and my partner when it potentially cost both of us our lives. Percocet from a past surgery, Ambien, and Xanax that he got that week. These were the pills scattered around us. I called three people—my neighbor, a doctor at the hospital and a very nice man, the attending that took him to strip clubs and showed him this lifestyle, and my friend. I said, "I need help. Don't call the ambulance." I was *still* protecting his livelihood, which had happened before.

All of us were physicians and he was coherent. I was like, don't do this to his record, just get him help. My friend came and helped me. My neighbor got the gun and showed me it was loaded, then it became more real. The other guy handed him a beer and told him to step outside to chat with him. You've got to be kidding me! Three times, I had wrestled the gun out of his hand, and this guy is handing him a beer.

We called his parents and they got on a flight that night. They stayed with him for a week. Only his father would speak to me. His mom blamed me. His dad whined, "What should we do? I don't know what to do. This is not my son." I told him, "This is your son. He has tried several times to commit suicide. I never called the ambulance, and I should have. You need to take him to the hospital. This is your son, it's your responsibility. I am no longer his partner. I have removed myself from this situation."

It took them a week to get admitted to a psychiatric ward. He was there for a week. They didn't get it. I should add that six months before this incident, going to the shooting range had become a hobby he had time for. It's normal where we live. I didn't like that he had bought a gun, but some of the doctors would take him to the range.

His dad informed me when he was in a psych ward. One day he was allowed to make calls. As if on cue, Paul called me from there and tried to apologize and also blamed me at the same time for this happening to him. That was the last time I spoke to him. He first said that he had learned so much then soon, he was trailing off into me having done something to him. Kind of like that phone call in the movies where it starts subtle and then someone trails into a completely different mindset. I didn't tell him where I lived, and he eventually found out and showed up several times.

I had to get a protective order against Paul. You have to buzz to get in the building and search my name. He would buzz and buzz and eventually, I had to give pictures to the security guards. Then he tried to run me off the road one day. He found me on the highway, going seventy-five or eighty miles an hour, and I was on my way to work. He must have been getting off the night shift because this was like 7:30 in the morning. Yes, he had gone back to work. The other doctors were protecting him. They gave him a couple of days of a leave of absence, and he flew to another city to see a friend and posted pictures of all the bars they were going to—while on medical leave. His parents allowed it, saying he just needed to get away.

We went to court a few times. I got the order extended. In the time I had thought it was extended and approved by the judge, he violated it by trying to hack into my email account, saying from Paul's iPhone. I gave the evidence to my lawyer. This was six months later. We went to court and what happened was he had dodged the subpoena, and his lawyer said, "If my client never received this, there is no protective order." The sheriff had not made sure he received it simply because "he's a doctor and works crazy hours." Meanwhile, he did get it because he wrote a letter to the judge saying he couldn't make the court date. My lawyer was livid. He was facing twenty days in jail and they couldn't arrest him. It backfired. The original protective order was for Paul trying to run me off the road. It was not a scare tactic. I've never seen the craziness in somebody's eyes so much as that day with him swerving, getting in front of me, slamming on his breaks.

He violated the order several times but escaped consequences using his title as a doctor. Simultaneously, he had done so much, and I had never filed a police report. Everyone was concerned about his livelihood. Nothing that had been in a paper trail could fully be considered. He told everyone at work what he did to me I did to him—that I tried to run him off the road, that he had a restraining order against me, which they all knew was false. For a while, people didn't know who to believe.

You look like the clear, level-headed one when the other person looks crazy, but because you're not telling anyone, someone else will tell the story to suit them. He made me look absolutely mad, hysterical. He told people I was locked up in a ward. I had just gotten a job with all this defamation around me. I didn't know half of what was being said until later. He was actively trying to hurt my practice and reputation. Everybody looked the other way and stayed away from me because they just didn't know.

I had friends of years who said, "Well, you're not the innocent type either." That was hard because I had tried to keep him afloat so many times and he was trying to ruin my career. This is an example of what psychology calls a smear campaign.

With all these instances involving the court, he got promoted to chief resident of his program and scored a fellowship of his choice. It wasn't just that there weren't repercussions; he was actually promoted while all this was happening. Now a lot of people dislike him as a person, but nobody of importance ever gave him repercussions for anything. There was no Mental Health Day for him.

CHAPTER 5

Bigger, Brighter Band-Aids

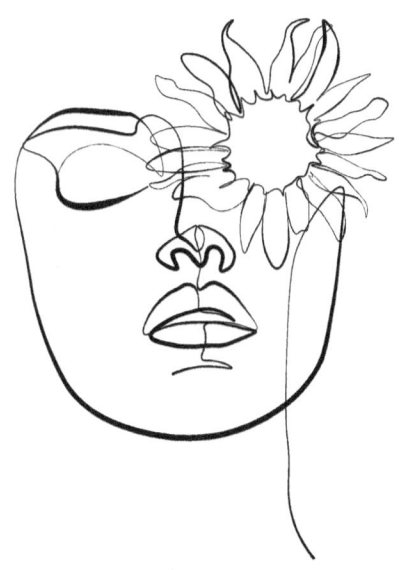

"We imagine that we want to escape our selfish and commonplace existence, but we cling desperately to our chains."

—Anne Sullivan

UNHEALTHY RESPONSES TO the intense stress that results from an abusive relationship have long-term effects on our health and stunt personal growth. In fact, responses such as overeating (to which I am an expert in as an obesity specialist), drug abuse, drinking, smoking, cutting, and many others, directly prolongs the vicious cycle of staying in an abusive relationship and can ultimately be fatal. Here are some of the most common:

Caffeine Overconsumption

It's important to note if you need caffeine to function or if you can go without it. This is a way to check your dependence on it. Cutting it off completely can result in rebound headaches and fatigue. Decrease consumption stepwise if you are choosing to do so. Caffeine in itself isn't harmful if you don't have anything such as a heart condition, so take this as general advice, not specific recommendations. Everything in moderation.

An occasional coffee is harmless but remember that caffeine has lasting effects on the body. Caffeine has an average half-life of five to six hours in the body of a healthy adult. It blunts the body's ability to absorb adenosine, a chemical that calms the body. Caffeine gives short-term alertness but causes sleep problems later on. It increases adrenaline and dopamine levels, resulting in feeling low after the initial high wears off, and could leave you agitated and edgy.

Fix: Pay attention to coffee's effects on your body and limit your intake. Avoid caffeine after 2:00 p.m. since it stays in your system for several hours and can disrupt sleep.

Compulsive Spending

There is nothing wrong with a little retail therapy in moderation. However, when we stress-shop, we are really looking for a dopamine hit. If it isn't in our budget or best interest at this moment, check in with yourself if you're seeking the item or the rush of the purchase. Dopamine can be obtained by exercise and nature as well, and these can be great substitutes when you feel the urge for a shopping spree beyond your means. A red flag is if you find yourself saying, "Oh, I'll make up for it next paycheck," as a justification.

Fix: If you can reduce your stress level, it's likely that you'll also reduce the likelihood of spending frivolously. Seek out one element of your life that you can let go of for a while. This may mean taking a personal day from work or letting the laundry go undone. Whatever it may be, step back and give yourself some breathing room.

Drinking Excessively

Alcohol dependence is another doorway to self-destruction. If you are using alcohol as a means to wind down and regularly, then it is by definition, becoming a coping mechanism. Alcohol should be moderately used for enjoyment, if you choose, but not as a coping mechanism. If you are drinking regularly, discuss with your physician ways to cut back safely. At certain levels, it is dangerous and even deadly to stop cold turkey.

While alcohol is related to stress-response dampening, long-term, heavy drinking can alter the brain's chemistry, resetting what is "normal." It causes the release of higher amounts of cortisol and adrenocorticotropic hormone. When this hormonal balance is shifted, it impacts the way the body perceives stress and how it responds to it. For example, a long-term heavy drinker may experience higher levels of anxiety when faced with a stressful situation than someone who never drinks or who drinks only moderately.

Fix: Limit alcohol to one drink per day. If you find that alcohol is your only way of regularly relieving stress, pursue other forms of stress relief.

Over- or Under-Eating

One in four Americans turn to food to help alleviate stress. People tend to fall into two appetite camps when stressed: craving carbs and sugar or a loss of appetite. While sugar can temporarily elevate your mood, glucose levels generally crash after two hours. Poor dietary choices lead to compromised health such as excessive weight gain, malnutrition, or chronic tiredness. Not eating enough is just as problematic, leading to fatigue, mood swings, and trouble focusing. It can also lead to diabetes, heart disease, high blood pressure and sleep apnea, to name a few.

Fix: Maintain stable blood sugar levels by eating a balanced breakfast, lunch, and dinner, with healthy snacking in between. If you're a grazer, carry protein-rich trail mix or granola bars, carrot sticks, edamame, or butter-less popcorn. If you lose your appetite, look to tension tamers such as yoga and journaling to help relax an anxious stomach. Don't be afraid to discuss your eating habits with your doctor and/or therapist. Together, these two approaches can make the world of difference in helping someone using food as a coping mechanism as it directly relates to morbidity and mortality. Sometimes a craving can be satisfied with a small piece of chocolate, hot tea, or allowing yourself some of what you want. The important thing is to recognize when you are having a craving and moderately allow yourself some without binging, and also not completely depriving yourself of foods. Deprivation leads to binging. If your mental health is suffering, address this first with professionals. You don't have to cope with anything alone.

Taking Medication, OTC or Prescription

Taking over-the-counter drugs like pain relievers, sleeping pills, and muscle relaxers when you're stressed out can often be like putting a bandage on a gaping wound; you might stem the flow a bit, but you need to go get stitches. OTC or prescription medication can temporarily relieve pain or anxiety and carries a risk of dependency.

Fix: Instead of chemical dependency, determine natural ways you can address symptoms of stress. Perhaps you're experiencing headaches because of a lack of sleep, or it may be time to visit your doctor. If you're having trouble sleeping or your muscles feel tense, opt for a good workout or a massage.

Poor Sleep

When it comes to sleep in times of stress, you can have too much (or too little) of a good thing. Where oversleeping is linked to health problems like diabetes and obesity, under-sleeping is linked to hyper-anxiety and memory loss.

Fix: The Sleep Foundation recommends sleeping between seven to nine hours a day. I always recommend using candlelight thirty minutes prior to bedtime. It's easier on the eyes and sets the stage for winding down. No electronics in the bedroom at all. Turn phone on silent and face down. Do not check the time if you wake up in the middle of the night; if your phone has an alarm set, you don't need to know what time it is. Take out all clocks in the bedroom, seeing that you have a phone with alarm. Any activities done prior to bed should be done in another room, so your brain is trained that the bed means it's time for sleep and not work.

Smoking

For smokers, a cigarette can feel like a good stress reliever. But while the cigarette industry's dwindling band of apologists claims that smoking relieves stress, a recent study found that smokers who quit were less anxious than before.

Fix: Talk to a doctor about medications that can help with smoking, and a plan to quit smoking long-term. Quitting cold turkey is also not recommended; it is best to have a plan and accountability along the way, as it is a true dependence. Quit-smoking programs are difficult, so when you feel like lighting up, seek support from family or friends, sharing your feelings and concerns openly. It's helpful to connect with someone who is quitting tobacco or has successfully kicked the habit long-term.

Overworking

Many people work as a way to not deal with their stress, but this will eventually backfire. If you find yourself picking up shifts and keeping busy, it doesn't always mean it's a bad thing but check in with yourself if it is sustainable. Everyone has different limits in this area. Give yourself permission to just be. If you think you can manage stress by working harder and more than normal, consider that overworked individuals tend to make more mistakes, which only leads to increased stress levels.

Fix: Work smarter, not harder. Take a break, have a nap, go for walk outside, and go back to spending time working as productively as you can.

Social Withdrawal

When we're feeling stressed, isolating in our comfortable beds for days seems like an attractive option. While some alone time is healthy, prolonged social withdrawal is a leading sign of depression.

Fix: It's okay to let your friends know you're struggling. Sometimes just a text is all you need to remember you aren't alone. Make social interaction a priority, as isolation can be harmful. We are social beings and thrive with some level of human interaction. Pets can also help in this area.

Not Dealing with It at All

Some of the best advice I was ever given is to allow myself to feel however I am feeling. If you need to cry, allow yourself. If you are angry, let yourself be angry. You don't have to take any action but sit with yourself and give yourself permission to feel whatever you are feeling. We often can't get to the analytical part with true clarity until we've allowed our feelings to be honored and present. Only then, we can rationalize what is going on underneath. Allow yourself to be human.

CHAPTER 6
In the Recovery Chair

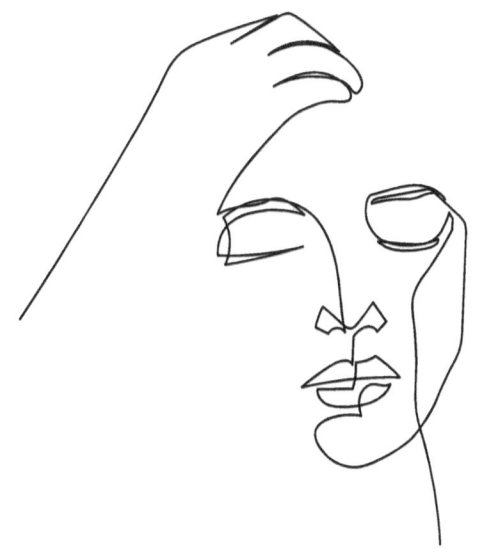

"Very often a change of self is needed
more than a change of scene."

—A.C. Benson

I EVENTUALLY LEFT MY job. I had had enough. I knew I couldn't work the way I was feeling every day, and I knew it would cost a practice and a community their doctor. That made me feel guilty, but I knew it was the right thing to do.

I actually spent five weeks abroad and took a legitimate hiatus. I ended up climbing Mt. Kilimanjaro with a friend, something I never thought I'd do: Hike the highest mountain in Africa and the highest single free-standing mountain in the world—with three volcanic cones, I might add. Not everyone has this luxury or even wherewithal to immerse herself in something like this, but it's a metaphor for how desperate and determined I was to reclaim my life. I had crawled on the floor at rock bottom and now, I needed to make my way to the top of my existence.

I took self-care to a new level for sure, but I absolutely needed to go halfway across the world to forget the pressures of work, the abuse of my ex, and the constant battle of trying to keep my head above water in my first real job. I came back with a completely new outlook, and my therapist had so much to do with helping me decide to live life differently.

Quora, an extensive online "spaces" forum on all topics imaginable, has 584,000 followers of the discussion board on the topic of "narcissistic personality disorder." Sample questions: Was the narcissist ever real or was it all a facade? Which side was the real him (sweet, affectionate, loving or pathological liar/gaslighter/cruel being)? Why do I feel I cannot love anymore after narcissistic abuse? The idea of a relationship repels me a lot. Why so? How do narcissists feel about the people who love them? Why, after a really good weekend with my ex-narcissist, is he now ignoring me all week and not replying? Do narcissistic fathers never listen to their adult children? Why do narcissists try and take your happiness and envy your confidence?

Conversations are a daily diet of disturbing experiences, but people are hungry for real answers about what they may be experiencing. As someone's narcissistic supply, you do a lot of second-guessing. It may go on forever without intervention.

Therapist Weatherly Camacho, LPC, agreed to share her expertise on narcissism, and I wish all 584,000 people on Quora and everywhere else with questions about what they may be experiencing could learn from her insights. I stand by the following dialogue, which reinforces all the stages I went through over the course of eight years and then in the aftermath. In order to keep the integrity of this valuable information, as she is a licensed professional, I offer it verbatim.

Q: *I'm hoping to capture an accurate depiction of narcissism from an expert point of view—what traits this condition is defined by and how it manifests in relationships (self and others).*

A: There are two types: *somatic*, grandiose like Paul, focused on financial gain and image; *covert*, meaning cerebral and sneaky. With narcissism at play, survivors get deeply entrenched in the abuse cycle, like when it's too late to prevent damage to themselves by the narcissist. They have an understanding but no registry of empathy, meaning they can exploit empathy, but they don't feel it. Narcissists will play mind games. For example, they will promise gifts but don't necessarily deliver on the promise. Their agenda is to damage the victim. Triangulation also occurs where they play two people off each other and make them compete for attention. They will also gaslight [meaning, sow seeds of doubt in a targeted individual or group, making them question their own memory, perception, or judgment]. They will complicate every situation.

They can't function otherwise, and they have an extraordinarily high IQ. There is also blame shifting, where feelings inside will be projected on the other person whether they did anything wrong or not.

Q: *Is abuse always an extension?*

A: Always, as it is part of a cycle with three primary stages. That person will adopt someone else's traits and goals to sell a future to the victim, and none of this is real. Future goals are shifted when they can't follow through. They need a narcissistic supply—every choice or promise is connected to ego avoiding responsibility and convincing the other person to progress in the "story." The deeper they are in, the more damage will be done, unfortunately. I have only dealt with one narcissist who I fully believe was aware of this without being told, fully aware of the damage and destruction he had caused, but only experienced guilt and shame after being exposed, with others knowing the truth of his actions. There is no turnaround here. They need a supply every way they can get it. There is always a body count of failed relationships. Lavishing emotions or berating the partner both fulfills them, and this is one of the most intense relationship roller coasters anyone can ever get on.

The stages:

1. Idealization stage or love bombing. They're charming, mirror your value system, and they're amazing and single! This stage is about securing the place to stay. They'll make comparisons between you and previous partners or parents, better or worse, so watch out for this. The victim is made to feel special and takes on every wrongdoing. They have a history of crazy people in their life exhibiting jealousy and

isolation. The covert one wants you to "have friends" but readily claims "our time together" separate from groups.

2. Devaluation stage, 9 to 21 months. The mask starts to fall and any weakness a victim exhibits, like fear of flying internationally and other human frailties that are normal, makes the victim a human being and inferior. Criticism comes and the person is intolerant of emotions and will start to distance themselves from the victim. This stage escalates tremendously, and they become abusive. The level of insecurity at this point seems unfathomable, treating the victim like garbage. Victim works harder and harder to bring back that ideal they once were to the point where they're becoming isolated from their support system.

3. Discarding, and this happens at the worst time, like the death of a parent, miscarriage, Christmas, or birthday, because they have another active supply. The victim questions their own reality and worth and turns on herself. Because they're so broken, suicide can even occur so the narcissist can play widow. If you've been married 10 to 15 years under these circumstances, the recovery period is much harder. No recollection of interests or who they really are because they've been stripped of identity. In therapy, we have to work to separate what they've been taught and what is healthy. They may even fear public spaces, panic, have emotional flashbacks because emotional neglect was prolonged. Here, we talk about cognitive dissonance. True success is the client moving forward from survival to thriving ("what happened to me" to "what happened for me"). Acceptance of all this shit comes from a wound in childhood typically. The narcissist pairs well with educated, empathetic people of a high standing, as it's the perfect challenge to chip away at their identity once they find a weakness.

In complete brokenness, there is no other place but healing. The victim must confront their inner being in order to live a healthy, happy life. It is mostly unconscious behavior, repeating their own toxicity from a parent.

When a narcissist can't attract supply, they become bitter and isolated. [Novelist and pioneer of the Beat Generation] Jack Kerouac is the perfect example of one.

They can put a victim on the shelf for years and then try to reestablish a relationship if they don't have supply.

A few other things: They are experts at removing boundaries and limits, which counters a healthy relationship. The partner literally loses self, loses reality. They're pushed into chaotic fights and beyond their limits. Once you receive a warning sign, reconnect with your boundaries and limits, or it's time to disconnect, period. True narcissists do not change.

And this is vital: 1. When a client has been around one, they all say, "We have a connection. He was watching me, adoring me from across the room." This is a shark studying prey. They're also extraordinary gift givers, tailoring to that prey. 2. Narcissists will repeat the same pattern from partner to partner, right down to where they go on vacation. They go with what they know and replicate. 3. Victims may be younger for more control. If they date the same age, the victim may be too wise. 4. Beware of emotionally withholding (sexually, silence, disappearances), stonewalling, and most psychological control, which is very abusive due to chaos and trauma bonding (being "addicted to this person" is a chemical experience).

What Makes the Perfect Supply?

Being called "supply" like a drug is demeaning in and of itself. But doctors are taught to use explicit language and ask patients to use explicit language to describe their ailments. It is in naming and calling it like it is that we can seek the appropriate solutions. So, again, what made me the perfect supply? Over the years, therapy has helped me pinpoint my history and use it to my advantage. You must know your story and be able to write the next chapter all on your own.

You simply cannot ignore your parents as major characters in your earlier story, even if they were not in your life.

My dad and I have a good relationship now, which I am thankful for, but his persona played a part in me being the perfect supply for a narcissist. As a cardiologist, when he started making money, the way he treated me and my mother at times was either buying us stuff or taking us on trips. If we disagreed with him over the weather, rain that day or not, he would be verbally or physically abusive. I remember him hitting me in the first or second grade. That was discipline, and he was disciplining his defiant child. I remember vividly it wasn't a pat on the butt; it was like that all-out loss of control and rage. He was going to keep doing it until he felt better, not to make a point or help me learn something.

I played a lot of sports. Once he realized I was really good at certain sports, he was set on me playing in college as the "best basketball player." At home, if I had a bad game, I would hear about it for days and days and days. It was a high-pressure home life with grades and sports.

My brother is four years younger and had the complete opposite experience from me. They were happy he graduated from high school. He's doing great with his life now. He's a people person. If I earned anything less than a B, all hell broke loose. With my brother, it was, "Please just get a C so we can move on." This was a small town, and everyone knew my dad. He took care of some family member of everyone's family. He needed us to uphold this image of a perfect family. My mother made a lot of excuses for his behavior. They would go to parties and act like everything was great, then at home, things were not. I grew up like that and ended up in a relationship with basically my dad. It backfired a lot worse in the end for me.

I had this reckoning as a teenager: this home life is not what it looks like in many other homes. I went away to college very far away for four years and didn't want them to talk to me. It's like I had to detox from this family system. I found myself and set out to do all these great things with my life, then I met Paul. I did not see it coming.

I am a lot more outspoken than my mom. She's more passive, but I am like her in the fact that I put others before me in a relationship or family. She would help me, but we wouldn't tell my dad. She took me to get my ears pierced. She taught me how to shave my legs. She wanted to help, but boys and sex were never topics. Catholic family, so all of that was tied to going to hell so let's not talk about it. This left a lot of burning questions.

My brother played football, baseball, lacrosse, everything my dad wanted in a son. Not book-smart and they worried about that. My brother is a graceful person. The way he was treated was completely different from me. He was male, and when he was in high school, my parents were separated and getting a divorce and I think they were so exhausted by each other they gave him what he wanted in terms of material things. We didn't have a close relationship growing up, but we've gotten closer since he got out of college.

Bodybuilding was something I could do all on my own without influence, instructions or demands. I could compete with myself and not have pressure of letting people down. My ex would say, "you look amazing," on some days, and on others, "you are such a cow, you shouldn't be on stage." He didn't come to my first competition. Any time something good happened, he would tear me down. My dad did a lot of things like that, too. He missed med school graduation and other significant events because there was always a fight or disagreement. Manipulators have to make everything about them. When I passed my boards, Paul did not attend, because he had to make the day about him.

Though he carried some of the same traits, Dad did not like Paul. We didn't speak for years. My dad called me about three and a half years after not speaking and he said he was sorry for the first time. He didn't want to die and never speak to me again. He felt like I wasn't going to chase after him anymore. I had been playing that card with him my whole life. I was still doing it with my ex. My dad's apology was the most genuine conversation I ever had with him and we've agreed to be friendly and still keep our distance a little bit, talking once or twice a month. I keep a lot of things private. I understand when he gives me little jabs, I have learned to just ignore. It's not worth fighting with him.

I told my mom about Paul's abuse and then my brother told my dad things I didn't want him to know. They both have concealed carrying licenses. On my graduation day of residency, they came down and they were carrying that night. They thought of him coming and making a scene. They were that worried after what had happened two weeks prior with the gun, that he actually would kill me that night. Maybe they were right. I don't think we all knew what he was capable of. They didn't tell me they were carrying. They didn't drink. They were there to celebrate me, which was really nice. I started to think, this must be more serious than what I think it is! When I started telling some of my friends of the physical abuse, they expected me to come apart in tears.

I've cried over it for sure, but it's easier to talk about than it should be. I experienced more embarrassment than anything. They all ask why I didn't say anything. Embarrassment sums it all up.

The girlfriend after me had contacted me asking if he had been abusive. When I had that conversation, she was ready to leave, then after a few days, I didn't hear from her. She then told me he threatened suicide if she left and "kept" her in the relationship. She eventually left and he never clearly followed through with it. I talked to my therapist a ton about this, but it's like he went to such a dark, deep level as a narcissist and in his depressed mind that he wanted to control everything. This wasn't just depression. It was another control method. He used information from his friend's suicide, seeing how much attention it had gotten, he kind of made it about him more than most people do. Narcissists make everything about them. They will take any event and make it about themselves. I have a lot of examples of that. I didn't realize it until after I left. When I took him back after the initial cheating, his parents looked at me like I was his medicine, the best thing for him. They said the same thing to the next girl, that he didn't need therapy or meds. This was their response to her crying out for help after an abusive incident. This was all him. His disorder also got worse as he got older. It typically peaks at twenty-nine or thirty years old. His other girlfriend called the police several times for choking her and stalking. Every relationship, it's a shorter time period of showing the bad side. By month three of four after love bombing, he might hit somebody. It gets shorter and shorter. I had the golden years of him in the early twenties before it really hit. That is why I stayed longer. What he is now, he was not ten years ago. He was developing.

My sense of guilt for staying—and even entering this relationship in the first place—often threatened to swallow me up if I did not completely heal from the abuse. Before you know it, you take in all blame as naturally as breath.

This has been a big part of therapy over months, that narcissists blame everything but themselves for the problem, especially when they have parents backing them up. I was always the problem or reason for him driven to this, whatever "this" was that day. When you're in it you don't see it for what it is. Once I learned he was exhibiting the same behavior with someone else, it set in that it was not me.

Pay attention to the following texts from the woman who got involved with Paul after me. How blindsided, how fearful, confused, isolated. It's also clear evidence that his behavior escalated:

"Was Paul abusive?"

"I have experienced both verbal and physical. It's unreal. He needs help."

"There's no way that behavior manifested overnight nor went unnoticed or experienced by anyone else."

"Hit, strangled, dragged by my hair, pushed in the shower."

"He literally bribes me not to work because he doesn't want guys to be around me without him around nor spending time apart. He's so controlling, it's unreal."

"When we were in France at 12:00 a.m. He openly strangled me on the street with people."

"In DC at a concert he got upset with me because I spoke up against some guys pushing into me. He started to belittle and insult me, so I ran away when the Uber arrived. He followed me to a neighborhood and choked me out. I screamed, lights came on, and he panicked. I hid behind a car because the police came. I got an Uber back to the Airbnb and slept on the couch."

"He has two guns now, but I don't know where they are. He threw his lithium away, too."

"He has literally put me in such a dark place I don't know who I am anymore. How could I let it get this bad? How didn't I see it?"

"I am too ashamed to tell my friends the full extent. ...I wish I would have taken pictures, but I am so tan only the worst bruises showed from when he pushed me in the shower. They lasted for days. You can tell people but without pictures, video, sound recordings, there's no real evidence."

"I think it started four, five months in with me. I'm an optimist and believer in people being good and changing if they truly try. My anxiety is through the roof."

"My friends worry, and they don't like him and never want to hang out with us."

CHAPTER 7
Grief is Not Depression

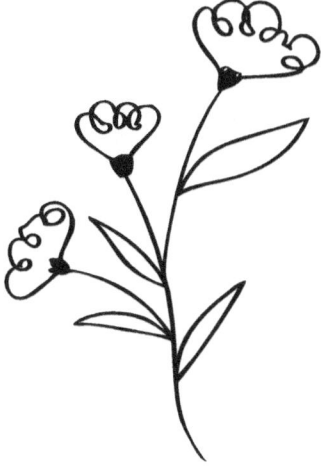

"I'm an emotional gangster. I cry once every month."

—Cardi B

You are put on a pedestal. If you like the color purple in the beginning of the relationship, they love the color purple. In the end, you find out they hate the color purple. They want to get you in their power and control.

How are you proofed from getting involved with a manipulator?

It happens in a gradual fashion, or it would be noticeable. It can start with criticism leading to an explosion if you don't follow the critique. It can range from the mundane, such as how to load the dishes, to how you talk to your friends (key: *your* friends). "Abuse" sounds like a strong word. The person can alter your own memories. Those who can provide high-grade narcissistic supply and those who cannot, who will be devalued and discarded. Narcissists feel empty inside, so they need other people to fill them up. It can be lots of different emotions, but they need to constantly extract some kind of emotion from you.

The abuse is detrimental to self-esteem because everything that was once important to you has been obliterated, piece by piece, like a solid block of ice chipped away into water droplets. They destroy your social network. You make big decisions because you think you're doing the right thing for the couple you have become, but they want you to be so invested, so trusted, that when they show you the monster, their true self, after exhausting their energy, you're stripped of faculties to deal with the aftermath or consequences of the decision. This could be as drastic as relocation. They may be damaged little children still, and their goal is to control someone else because they are incapable of becoming whole. They put on a convincing show of affection and love. Until you are dependent socially, mentally, financially perhaps. They need you in a weakened state to have influence. There is no functioning conscience.

Most psychopaths never go to jail. They just walk amongst us.

And this is where you have to fully focus on your own life—not where they are or what they are doing. It's time to grieve. Practice self-compassion. Extend the same compassion to yourself that you do when your friends are down on themselves.

Regular cycles of grief apply to death of relationships, death of dreams.

The difference between what people perceived as depression in me was that it was grief. I had a lot of grief after the relationship ended, mostly about losing myself and realizing I didn't know who I was anymore—not grief over loss of the ex. It felt like the death of myself, which happened over years but the realization of it was the worst and hit me like a bag of bricks. I had devoted so much time focusing on him that I hadn't taken care of myself at all. I questioned everything I ever did or said I wanted, or said I liked, not knowing if I did or if he did and manipulated me.

Many people do not realize this, and brush it off as, "Oh, she's depressed because of the breakup," but it's so much deeper than that. You realize you don't know yourself anymore. It's a scary feeling! People sense sadness and relate it to me canceling a wedding or breaking up with my fiancé. People kept telling me to "try medication" but grief is normal and necessary even though it hurts. In fact, that was the biggest relief I had ever felt. It felt like freedom from jail or like I was given a new life.

If an episode of "Grey's Anatomy," when Christina Yang didn't walk down the aisle to marry Dr. Burke, she ripped off her wedding dress because she felt so claustrophobic by the relationship. This gives you a good idea of what that felt like. Visuals help me to explain things!

I remember crying at times in my new apartment and smiling so big at the same time—such a crazy feeling to be grieving and so happy. I felt kind of crazy, but it was very real and intense having a strong sense of liberation for the first time in my life.

CHAPTER 8
The Bridge for Discontented Doctors

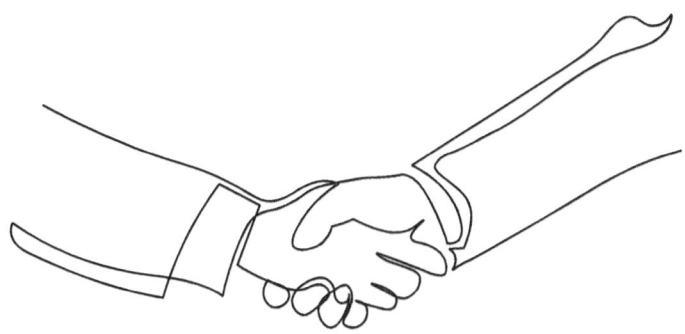

"Vulnerability is the birthplace of connection and the path to the feeling of worthiness. If it doesn't feel vulnerable, the sharing is probably not constructive."

—Brené Brown

Self-Care RX

DOCTORS NEED SELF-CARE, too. Remember, people turned a blind eye when Paul displayed erratic behavior. His whole success model was built around not admitting mental illness. It's really important. Suicide is prevalent in the military and medical industries. People in the military world do branded runs and awareness campaigns, but among physicians, mental illness is not talked about.

In Dawn's view, "A lot of physicians do have emotions that they don't show because everyone just thinks they are resilient. I compartmentalize a lot of things, put my emotions in the back of my head and keep going through the day, I can see when people don't know how to cope. Physicians don't ask for help, but more so, people don't think they need help because they are physicians. They don't think there is any reason to be depressed. No. 1 reason for being depressed is finances and since everyone thinks they are rich, there is no reason. Personally if I am having a bad day, talking to my family is just not in the question because I am the one to call if they are having a bad day. Forget about my bad day! I don't mind but that's just how it is. They don't think I'm capable of having a bad or sad day. They think I don't have problems because I'm too busy. Doctors don't get help and when they do have signs, people don't acknowledge them. Our own humanity is kind of being ignored sometimes. A lot of doctors alienate themselves, too. Most of us have friends and family to talk to, but certain few are alienated. They go home and live alone. They have higher divorce rates because they work a lot. All of that stuff is just going to make you depressed."

"With one completed suicide every day, US physicians have the highest suicide rate of any profession," reported *Medscape Medical News*, citing research in 2018. "In addition, the number of physician suicides is more than twice that of the general population."

There is so much pressure in that field that if you are viewed as someone with a mental health issue, you can't go save someone else's life if you have trouble yourself. With Paul, his family always attributed blame to someone or something else, not him. There were so many things I hid for that fear of his career. I didn't even question if I was doing the wrong thing until it got so bad for me. I had basically enabled him to abuse me by protecting his interests.

I alerted who I thought would care the most, like his brother and some people that we worked with. Everyone wanted to turn a blind eye. It was a hard spot for me to be in, to go above the people that were closer to him. It would be like a disciplinary action. I was scared. Particularly for someone who didn't want to help, it put me in a position. That is the norm of the environment. Even as a physician, I didn't question if I was doing the wrong thing.

There is a key portion that is different about this person. I'm still not sure if bipolar was the correct diagnosis. He is 100 percent a full-blown narcissist. People throw around traits that could be related. But everything they do is for attention in some way. I look back at when I left that relationship, I thought I was letting someone down who could potentially commit suicide one day. The more I learned about what happened, I realized that every move, every phase, was toward keeping me in the relationship, which is a scary topic. When his friend had committed suicide, it's almost like he took the idea and then from that point on, decided that was what he would use every time I would try to leave or confront the relationship issues. It was a really tricky situation. I didn't really know if he would commit suicide or this was something he was saying. You don't want to chance the alternative. When I came home that day and he was on the bed with the gun and the letter, the bed had been made. It wasn't like he was in the center of a messy room, wrestling with the meaning of life. It was almost like he heard me coming and laid on the perfectly made bed deliberately.

Dr. Pamela Wible writes and speaks about physician suicide. She is very passionate about this particular issue and knew many physicians who committed suicide during her training, sparking her determination to speak out and use her voice as influence. Perhaps her most important effort has been assembling the book, *Physician Suicide Letters Answered*. You may already cringe at this topic, raw to the bone, but believe me, "what you don't know about medical training and culture can kill you," as stated in the synopsis. There is a "pervasive and largely hidden medical culture of bullying, hazing, and abuse that claims the lives of countless medical students, doctors, and patients."

When I started my new job at age thirty, I found myself more compassionate towards people that were going through a hard time in life much more easefully than before. I could understand real pain, whether it was someone going through a divorce or in a toxic situation. There was no "suck it up" mentality anymore; my younger self might have thought this. I won't lie.

Asking about people's mental health became more of a priority but was tough because it's a time-consuming topic in a busy primary care office. Focusing on obesity, I realized how many people suffered from some type of toxic situation from someone else or themselves. The toxic ingredient wasn't simply sugar. It could be a relationship, poor self-esteem, unchecked intergenerational trauma or a recent traumatic situation. The way we talk to ourselves is so important, and the majority of people don't know how to properly self-reflect. Many people do not want to go to therapy because of time or money, but in reality, it's the best thing for them.

What I also found from my own struggles starting a job amidst all of this chaos in my own life was that I had a tough time mentally focusing on so many patients in need. I wasn't okay myself, yet I was trying to take care of thousands of patients. I became very irritated easily, especially with the demand from patients in healthcare today. No one likes to wait at the doctor's office; every person wants to speak to the doctor directly during the workday (at least now, chat is more prevalent), and twenty-four hours seems too long to wait for lab results when there would be 100 of them for me to respond to. I needed a break, and I was just starting my career.

I should have been that bright-eyed new graduate everyone thought I was, but I needed a hiatus from life in general. It's really tough when so many people depend on you to put yourself first. I had to learn quickly to say no to more patients, extra hours, extra responsibilities. I want to be the person that can help anyone that needed it, but I was out of gas for sure.

The morning that Paul tried to run me off the road, I called police as soon as I got to work and told my office manager. Soon after I obtained a good behavior order from the court system, which really didn't help. He was never arrested. I went into work and saw patients regularly that day, mentally a mess, yet not able to take a day off for my own mental health.

He ended up telling people around the hospital that I ran him off the road and I was crazy. It's easy to see how a physician can start to lose compassion when they are running on empty. Whenever I hear "horror" stories from patients or the gen pop about horrible doctor bedside manner, I often question to myself what that person may be struggling with. I have a much different perspective of jaded physicians. Most of the time, I just see pain, burnout, and depression. This isn't to say I excuse it, but I understand it. It's why I started coaching physicians about self-care. I was there myself, and I consider myself an empathetic person. If I could lose capacity for human interaction, so can anyone else under the right circumstances.

I scanned every car every time I drove to work from that point on. At every restaurant I walked into, I had to sit facing the open room. Every time I walked downtown, I had to basically keep a look out. There was no real relaxation, no break. I felt haunted by what might happen at any moment. And there were zero repercussions for him. For me, the repercussions were a constant state of fear and my mental and physical health deteriorated, which ultimately is their goal.

To me, lack of self-care is the issue in my profession. I have no issue working twenty-four hours straight because I am in a healthy place mentally to do so. I've done it in unhealthy mental states in which I didn't care as much. Life outside of work was too bleak and exhausting. Sadly, we go into this to take care of people, but no one is looking out for physicians' well-being. We are viewed as unstoppable superhuman creatures and that's pressure enough to where people don't speak up or take time they need. I've learned the best way to be selfless is to actually be selfish first, then you have the energy to give back compassionately.

Giving Back on Common Ground

One of my newfound good friends, who I will call "Joanna" to conceal her identity, is from a mastermind I joined. I met some amazing people and all with tremendous stories of hitting rock bottom and doing their own thing. I talked to this woman whose ex was a narcissist and she's in a stalking situation as of this writing. Her situation has been volatile. The severity of it reinforces that these people are everywhere! She was in pharma for twelve years in executive positions. She endured bullying in the workplace and then at home. Her first narcissistic ex was a covert narcissist—he was secretive and highly manipulative. She ended up leaving her corporate job while in the mastermind to work on her own self-care and leadership skills while coaching others on how to be a leader while putting yourself first. We call her the CEO whisperer! You have all these executive-level women who, in the workplace, are not allowed to be human or feminine or caring or beautiful, without another compromise or cost. Who she is emits such light and amazing energy.

Still, she fell back in another relationship via love bombing. There were a lot of lies and secret drug use. After wooing her, he broke objects and punched her television, stalked her across state lines, threatened the lives of her parents if she didn't meet him in an alley in the middle of the night to talk. Then he abused their pet to the point of almost killing it.

She shares her story, which is occurring in the here and now: "People can empathize, but unless you have been in this situation, you can't really understand. Danielle was my rock. She was my beautiful, successful friend who you would never think this could happen to. She was my mirror to say, this *can* happen to you. You didn't do anything wrong, and you will get through this. There were times when I just wanted to keep the dog safe and let everything else go. She insisted, 'But that is not the path. It feels easier, but then you have no recourse. He will never stop.' She helped me on the days I could barely function. She reminded me I didn't have to work eighty hours a week. I could take the day off. Managing this is a fulltime job.

"Who was this person before all came to light? I met him at the gym. Incredibly charismatic charmer. Good-looking guy. He was 'honest' with me the first time we hung out that he had an explosive separation from his ex, there had been a restraining order. He broke the order trying to talk to her. That he had been to jail, but he had a well-crafted victim story. It was a fifteen-year relationship that went on seven years too long. He was the victim. He was being honest and transparent. I felt like I was really special because he had been so vulnerable with me. He was very good at studying what I wanted, and he was able to portray this person I wanted for about three months. It became very difficult to keep up this façade. He had no real friends and a rocky relationship with his mother. He had just moved to town, and some of the guys at the gym liked him. Then he started walking back from the dreams and plans we made: 'I don't want to be around people.' 'I don't want to host dinner parties.' 'I don't want to move to California,' which is where we talked about moving together. He was only making a third of the money he claimed and was having financial challenges. It started to crumble. We took a break in fall. I had taken him to a family wedding and my family loved him. We were taking a walk and he just lost it on me. We were supposed to be at a family function, and he disappeared, wasn't answering his phone. I told him after that occasion, you have a lot to figure out. I can't do this.

"Fall of 2019, I had seen him in the gym one night that I didn't feel well. He said, 'I would love to buy you soup', but he didn't have his wallet. I wanted chicken noodle soup and couldn't find any and texted him this story. He didn't respond, which was weird. Next day, I looked on his mom's Facebook page. He had been hit by a drunk driver while helping a friend move. He was injured badly and lived in a walkup, so I offered to take care of him at my place. I nursed him back to health. I didn't know he was taking steroids because he didn't want to lose muscle while he was injured. That was my first taste of his rage cycles. It was mostly blackmail-manipulation. I was going on a retreat to California, and he would record our calls because he didn't like that it was a co-ed retreat. He got me to talk about different guys at the retreat and threatened to send them the recording. He buys phone numbers and uses them to harass people. He has used so many numbers to call me that they can't trace it. Our municipal police forces don't have the resources to do that.

"I let him back into my life because he was in church and counseling. We were always together in the pandemic. Stephan wanted to get this special breed of dog and they need so much structure. He knows his rules, but he doesn't care. It made Stephan fall apart. He started using steroids again. In the summer, he decided to move to South Carolina because I wasn't going to have him, a rare puppy, my dog and my cat all working from home in a one-bedroom loft. On July 4th weekend, we had a wonderful weekend. Our agreement was for me to take care of all the animals until he got settled in South Carolina. I left the puppy there and within twenty-eight hours, he tried to kill him, Facetimed me. I knew immediately something was wrong. I said, show me 'Furry'. He was in a corner as far away as possible hyperventilating. He had hung Furry and went into another room until he couldn't hear movement. He had only passed out, thank God. When he came back in and took the dog down, he started breathing again. Danielle and I have a common therapist. She said it is sociopathic. He doesn't have the courage to see consequences. He threatens my family's safety. He didn't want to see the dog die, but he took the direct actions that would lead to it.

"I went to get the dog and my intention was to get him to sign over the dog. Stephan owed me $7,000, and soon, I was able to get him to sign over the dog and I would forgive his debt. When I started enforcing the boundary, two weeks later maybe, when he wanted the dog to come and stay with him, shit got nuts. He stalked me, filed a false police report to the tune of the officer screaming in my face and then apologizing via my attorney because of the story Stephan had convinced him of. He is a master manipulator. Then he had COVID and other supposed issues.

"When I got a restraining order, I was really scared and stayed in a hotel. He had been sharing location with me on the phone and we were in the same state. Then he was sending me erratic texts: *I've never loved you. If anything, I've hated you.* I had already sought legal help in order to keep the dog safe. He told me to get out of my house and go to a hotel for the weekend. I was voice-messaging

Danielle on Sunday when I went back home and Stephan called me twice, then called me from a blocked number and then texted me and said, 'I just saw you leave your place. You have to give me the dog. The police are here.' I called 9-1-1 and they said no one had been dispatched. I have text messages of the night he tried to kill the dog. He had written, 'He is sleeping on my lap, even though I tried to end his life, he can love me unconditionally.' I have so much evidence. Along the way, he had talked about his ex like, 'I dream of standing over her dead corpse. I am going to burn the barn her sister is getting married in.' He was able to layer that in such that I am terrified he is going to do something to me. The dog stuff, the texts about his ex and stalking me, that is why I got the restraining order.

"We are tied up in the middle of litigation, criminal charges. One, he is suing me to get back a dog he tried to kill. He sent Danielle a video just yesterday through her website submission that he wanted me to see. He was addressing me. It's like the proverbial frog and water. I was in this pan of water and the temperature was getting turned up so slowly that I didn't know what was happening around me until I was burning. This foundation for manipulation, for abuse was made ever so slowly. I was tired, having energy drains but I didn't realize the magnitude of manipulation and abuse until he tried to kill the dog. I upended my life. I'm on another coast now, awaiting some sign that I can get on with my life again in a permanent home. I spent a lot of time with Danielle. I look at this whole thing as a blessing. For the first time in my life, I had to accept help from people. She never asked me when I was leaving. I'm not able to live peacefully.

"I've done a lot of inner work and therapy to now know I have a pattern of abandoning myself to love and that stems from my mother. My parents divorced when I was four and I carried all of her worries. I existed to serve her first and then me. I wasn't learning the lesson, so I needed Stephan to show me these patterns. My mother controlled me through fear. She was so afraid something would happen to me, but it wasn't me, it was because of how *she felt*. That is a pattern that repeated with Stephan in a big way. Stephan preyed on that vulnerability. I would capitulate when he would threaten to bring in other people. He contacted my ex-husband. I never wanted to bring drama to other people. This all ties back to a childhood pattern that I hadn't woken up to before therapy. I have complex PTSD in which when something with Stephan happens, I flash back to childhood. I took on other people's pain. I carry so much of his pain.

"I had to upload a video yesterday for the district attorney that took four hours. Thank god I am an entrepreneur and can set my own schedule. Danielle was my strength some days. I stayed with her and I was protected by her. She put herself out there and risked her safety. Danielle's biggest strength was the constant reminder that I didn't do anything wrong. I would see him after the restraining order and she would be in my ear, saying call the police. It sounds weird but it was scary for me to call 9-1-1. I had never called the police before last year. This is so far removed from how I live my life. To have a friend who was equally successful, talented, who was in a worse situation candidly and now has a beautiful partnership, and was able to thrive, she was my hope. She was exactly like me and that was everything. You think of women with kids, lower socioeconomic status. I put up a video on Instagram when it was happening and the number of women who were just like us—that this happened to them, it was mind-blowing. We're the perfect archetype. We work really hard. We're fixers. We fight hard for things.

"Right from growing up, I was used to something very chaotic. It felt familiar. I've had a couple of interactions with other guys. But if it's not fireworks, am I into him? Do I like him? I don't know. This is why we have therapy. With Stephan, there was something so similar energetically, but then when we got to this point, it's so far from how I live my life. There is something called the 'sociopathic stare'. I remember being keenly aware of Stephan the very first time I saw him in the gym. He said he always knew where I was in the gym. They target you and they watch you. I mistook that for butterflies, a karmic connection. My body was giving me alarm bells instead. It's happened since and I could not get far enough. Another time, I looked at a guy like seven times and his energy was the same as Stephan's. It felt so terrifying whereas before, it felt exciting. I misunderstood what it was."

I want to point out something very unique in Joanne's narrative here that is rarely discussed in terms of chemistry. Contemplate if you have experienced this. It may answer a lot of questions and help you shift patterns. That spark, electricity and energy. We know all too well what that is. The point she made about us being opposite sides of the same coin energetically and mistaking danger for butterflies is huge! I had the same realization through my therapy. It's the first sign our body is trying to tell us to run away to safety, but we never knew safety to begin with. This also speaks to our success in the workplace of making sure we are safe in an almost overcompensated way.

I think it's common in general and it's a spectrum like anything else. The narcissist being the polar opposite of an empath energetically is chilling, because they are equally as intuitive, but their intentions are sadistic/healing respectively.

Joanne is thirty-eight years old, successful, attractive, well-informed, and self-aware, but there is a lot internally that could continue to be harmful. "I see that my greatest love is on the other side of this. Without waking up to these patterns and wounds and truly healing co-dependency, I could never enter that partnership in a healthy way. I took a long time to understand what was holding me back. I wish I could stop carrying the 200-pound weight and have the greatest partner, be a mother. I feel it and I believe I will have all of those things. I know it's there for me. It's partially my age and experience, but it's been discipline and the disposition I have carried since my divorce in 2017. I have a daily gratitude practice and I never let that waver. I choose to take responsibility for my part in this. He didn't just pick me. There were things I was attracted to and I take responsibility. I see it as a lesson. I see this man as incredibly broken who needs so much help. I want him to face the consequences and I want to be safe. I want other women safe. There are few moments I'm like woe is me, I don't live there. I have a low tolerance for people who use substance or other mechanisms to avoid their emotions. I have to leave. I get very uncomfortable and have to leave. I'm growing. It's been a discovery for me being there for someone else who is going through this."

We have to get to know ourselves and why we keep choosing these patterns. Her mother was codependent. She looked to Joanna to soothe her needs starting at the age of four. She became a problem solver for people's hardships. Learning how to not be so giving is hard. This is Joanne's self-discovery journey. The intent is never bad. A parent can ingrain a certain behavior in you. You learn when you get older it's not working for you!

She had to get a new phone, new car. He used fake numbers to call and track her. He used social media to create fake accounts as her characterizing her as a drug addict to try to tarnish her reputation. By the way, this is very hard to convict someone of. I had endured a decent amount of defamation, or cyber libel, and I learned that knowing the law and your rights is a form of self-care.

According to Traverse Legal, in order for a comment, post or article to constitute internet libel, the following elements must typically be met:

- The first thing you must prove is that the statement constitutes a false statement of fact. A fact is different than an opinion. A fact can be proven true or false. Opinions are typically not actionable as defamation.

- The false statement of fact must harm your reputation. There are many false statements posted across the internet. In order to constitute libel, a statement must not only be false but must harm you or your company's reputation and cause harm.

- The false statement of fact causing harm must be made without adequate due diligence or research into the truthfulness of the statement. Alternatively, plaintiffs often attempt to prove that the false statement of fact was made with full knowledge of its falsity.

- If the person who is the subject of the false statement of fact is a celebrity or public official, the plaintiff must also prove "malice." Malice is proven when the person posting the information on the internet intended to do harm or acted with reckless disregard of the truth in making the statements.

The Internet is such a big part of Joanne's trauma story because she is an entrepreneur online. Social media was her marketing. Watching her endure that while she was growing her business was hard to see because the court system had no way of verifying these things. Of course, she knew it was him. This type of person is so obsessed with ruining you that they will stay up all hours of the night with an endless energy to come after you until they are satisfied.

CHAPTER 9

Whole, Healed, Remembered

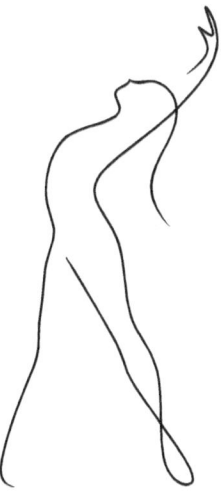

"When it comes to our collective health, how we deal with the multiple crises and problems around us also depends on the power of context—in other words, our resilience."

—Arianna Huffington

Self-Care RX

Diana Guy, who I consider a self-care warrior, is nearing her fiftieth anniversary of practicing and teaching Hatha yoga and meditation—I feel very fortunate to be able to share her story in *Self-Care Rx*. In 1973, her initial entry into yoga was a "night out," but no one knew of the nightmare she was experiencing at home when she started. Though we come from vastly different generations, her story really resonates with me.

Legendary Lilias Folan, an icon on TV at that time, was teaching yoga with relaxation being a major focus. Relaxation was a profound concept for Diana. Out of sixty-five people in the class that night, she was sure she was the only one having chaotic half-sentences in her head. She was so anxious, which she had not noticed before. Her twenty-three-year-old body was so stiff and sore. Realizing all this was so sad to her psyche and body at this young age. But if I think of where I was at the same age, well, I don't want to think about it either. Instead of running from that anxiety, Diana looked at it and decided to go back each week for a ten-week session. She journaled about her experience and reactions to yoga and relaxation. Lilias became Diana's mentor and encouraged her to study in-depth with her teachers and friends at a yoga seminary in New York. Then Diana began traveling with her and teaching, subbing for her and offering her own classes and workshops. In 1975, Diana and other teachers began the Cincinnati Yoga Association, which is still one of the largest in the world. For all the masses Diana has taught, touching every walk of life in almost fifty years, it's astounding to hear that she once had no real reference for self-worth, self-care. This vulnerability led her into an abusive marriage.

"Our parents had the 'man-superior and authority toward women' instinct in that generation. Coming from that and then in the sixties, that attitude was revolted against and women began shifting into their own power. That shift is really important. Having said that about the generation, in Jim's family, it was not his father. It was his mother with a strong personality, which often was negative, and his father was soft-spoken, gentle and quiet. With Jim being the youngest, his mother spoiled him. Different behavior traits like his terrible temper were often overlooked and never addressed. When we met in high school in the sixties, I was a teenage girl receiving attention and gifts and hanging out with this cool guy in a cool car. Alcohol was involved and there were early expressions of lack of respect, like putting me down or not showing up on time. I left him then because that continued to escalate. I dated other men and one in particular, Ken, who was so kind, fun and had so much depth. Jim knew I was dating others, so he came back in the picture with more gifts and promises—like marriage. That paralleled at the time with my mother seriously ill and dying. My desire was to give my mother a wedding. I married Jim.

"On the day of my wedding as we were getting in the car with my dad, my mother said, 'If you do not want to go through with this, we can take you to the airport.' She must have seen signs of discontent. Once in the marriage, the drinking worsened, and physical abuse began. I was pregnant with my daughter. His brother came to get me out of the abuse one time and took me to their house. Jim's mother saw my bruises and said, 'Well, there's another side to this story,' so I may have deserved it. He would apologize and I would get back with him. This continued. Then we built a home. By then, the three kids were born. My son was nine months old when I started yoga with a group of women, off to take Lilias's class. I still have my journal of that progress in my class. I was ninety-eight pounds, just lifeless with these three kids. As I became more deeply interested and practiced daily, my changing in a healthy way and into my own power threatened Jim. He became promiscuous. I never knew when he was coming home day or night. We did agree to a separation. Then during the separation, he escalated, threatening me with guns. It got worse and worse. The restraining orders never worked. I had a wonderful support system of women and men from my holistic community who helped me many times. I remember being on the phone crouched under a chair because I was afraid that he was going to come with a gun and shoot me through the window. Now, would he have killed me? I think so at some point, but the whole thing of holding you in fear is a high for these abusers. That is their power over you. He knew that with my studies and my practice, I was changing and seeing him more clearly. I was receiving different ways of being, even with men. Yoga was the root of my self-worth and I went every day to generate that energy as his behavior continued to escalate.

"One evening in front of the kids, he had a shotgun and was going to shoot me. My daughter managed to step away and call my friends, a mother and daughter. The mother talked him down while the daughter helped me prepare to leave. I left barefoot out the door and never returned. That was my last time in that house. In another scene, at the airport, I was with a Christian mystic. We had to leave Grailville, a holistic retreat center, because he was coming there to shoot me. She and I went to Florida, her place, and he actually jumped on a plane after us. She did not let me go to meet with him at the airport. He handed over the gun to her and her husband. He had stopped drinking because he had a bad car accident. Yet still this behavior. It never stopped. I know I had PTSD, but it wasn't called that at the time. Even though we had been divorced for so many years and we both remarried, every time I would see him, there would be fear and held breath. Still, I turned my whole yoga practice into helping others with addiction, depression, new ways of being calm and interacting. Relaxation was my specialty, and I was awarded Holistic Women of the Year from *New*

Life magazine. There is no doubt in my mind if I didn't have that world, I would not exist—either through my own depression or him doing me in. Until his death, I always had a sense of mistrust. He would appear on my doorstep or have an angry expression at the children's events.

"It was subtle. It was disrespect. Then we didn't have cell phones so I would never know when he was coming. Then verbal. Then it became pushing. He would say in court and to the therapist, 'I never hit her, I just pushed her.' It escalated to the threat to kill me and then to taunt me. He would be somewhere on a pay phone saying stuff. If we had cell phones, he could have tracked me. When we got married, he had me in a house in containment. Now, Jim was not a narcissist, but abuse is abuse. The survivor of a deep level of abuse responds and reacts in a similar way. You're losing yourself. Five years into all this, I began yoga. I had a new house, three kids, what may have looked successful on the outside, but it was draining every which way.

"The boys don't remember, but my daughter does. Had I stayed in that, it would have been imprinted in the boys' behavior possibly, but they are such gentle, heart-centered creatures—all of my kids. On his death bed, he apologized, but it took him that to let go. The drugs were able to relax him so he could not maintain that posture of anger. Isn't that interesting? My sense is he probably was bipolar or some undiagnosed mental condition. He never had a life after I left him. He and his other wife did nothing, no social interaction with people. I'm grateful that he was able to say the words, but I told him that it was all healed; to move on with death and dying. After he died, I could finally do this deep sigh. I didn't realize I lived in sporadic held breath for so many years.

"Here is the thread in all of this regarding depression and the suicide rates. Those components are within. The cancer group, who have been diagnosed, the families who are caretakers to drug addicts, to people who are abused, and prenatal—the anxiety, fears, drama or any trauma—accident or self-imposed, all of that is woven into any of these groups. What the yoga and meditation is able to do is gently start to release where that is held in the body, start to release the held breath. As I always say, we hold our breath more than we breathe, and we don't realize that. YOU MUST BEGIN RELEASING THE BREATH. In a class, it's more subtle. In a private session, the results are more dramatic because you can really dive into the individual experience. Hormonal imbalance is also a symptom that is helped. Without self-care, we are lacking a sense of intimacy within ourselves and love for ourselves. I studied this in the eighties. Here we are in 2021, and we live in a great deal of staccato rhythm. We become filled with tension and anxiety and we don't realize it. It's our norm! Thus, the suicide rates. We get in a chaotic mess and we don't know how to deal with it, so that is our way out. Look at our news cycle. It keeps us in a state of flux of chaos. Everyone needs to work on themselves—at any time. To me, there is no better way to do it than yoga. It integrates the body with the mind and the heart and spirit. It's all-encompassing. It can be so simple when it is taught properly. Then you reap the benefits of it. Breath alone is a powerful place to begin to shift into change and get into your own power."

CHAPTER 10
Don't Hold Your Breath

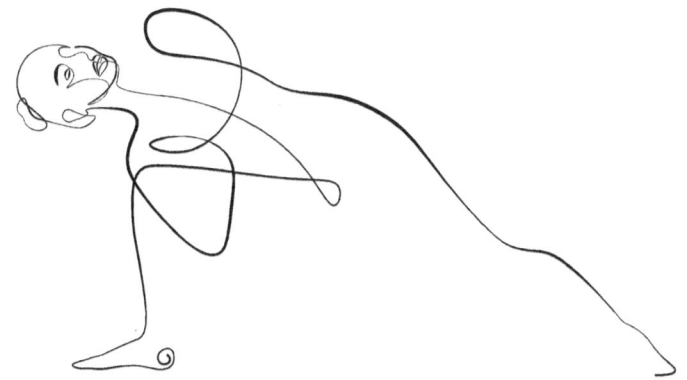

*"Ultimately we know deeply that the
other side of every fear is freedom."*

—Marilyn Ferguson

Self-Care RX

I LOVE DIANA'S STORY and I'm so thankful she and her children are safe and thriving! I understand what she means about holding your breath, or never being relaxed because abusers like to hold fear of unexpected actions over you constantly. My friend, Dawn, told me after my relationship ended that I was a visibly anxious person from the day she met me. I had no idea I was this way. I didn't know what relaxation was. Even my vacations would be jam-packed with things to do because of the risk of my ex being "bored" or it wasn't the "most impressive trip ever." Learning how to breathe in yoga made me feel different. I didn't know why at the time. It makes perfect sense. In yoga, you are left to be with your own breath, which is ironic and profound to say!

Dawn got me into yoga mostly for fun exercise, but it actually became a very therapeutic too. There were times I would be in yoga and cry freely. It forced me to be in my own thoughts, my own body. It's amazing how much we can suppress and never realize it, and still be high functioning. I've been an athlete my whole life, competitively and for fun, and there are days I *need* yoga. Some people may feel that way about running or something else, but yoga allowed me to self-reflect in a way that I didn't know how. It was the thing I didn't know I needed.

My ex currently lives on the other side of the country, and I can't say I feel relieved. That fear they hold over you, especially with social media these days, never truly leaves—it's learned and programmed. It is very difficult to release yourself from what you know they are capable of. I know the day I left him, I said out loud, "I'm going to die in this relationship." It wasn't that day, but I knew it was possible. Diana seemed only to have felt safe with her ex-husband's death. That's powerful and I completely understand why.

I've only recently begun to identify with being a survivor. This didn't click for the longest time, even though my therapist incessantly stressed I was a survivor. It clicked even more when I sat next to a woman on a plane who lost her daughter because her boyfriend stabbed her to death. She was flying to Chicago to pick up her daughter's body. I had a panic attack when I got off the plane. My boyfriend at the time had struck up a conversation with her, then told me later in the flight her story. It felt close to home. I wanted to hug her so hard.

We might see these stories on "Dateline," but we don't usually know who of our own friends or acquaintances might be a potential victim.

I remember being in court a few years ago because Paul refused to leave me alone. I had to move twice and get a new car to try to hide from him. He did not stop stalking me. I was seeing a man at the time, who showed me a normal relationship and great compassion for what I was going through. Our intimacy didn't rely on chaos. He cared about my interests, my feelings. He was protective, and I will forever be grateful that he was there for me during that time. We had been dating a couple of months and he called me one night after watching a "Dateline" episode featuring the story of an ex-boyfriend killing this girl after she had moved on. He insisted, "You need to move. You need to get away…please," since Paul had been showing up every few months completely unstable. I was out of touch. I was so used to his craziness.

Whether a real threat or not, Paul did threaten to kill me. You never think that somebody is going to kill himself or kill you, and that is how these stories end up playing out. It took a while for me to realize the severity. I wasn't going to the gym or running outside because I was so scared to be seen. I was showing it, but I was not feeling it—I was very numb.

I held it together so well for years. I have moments here when I feel vulnerable and go back and forth between wanting to put this book out there to help people, to wow, I suck for putting up with this for eight years. Then when I think of a few people who interrogated me rather than showed that they cared for my wellbeing, I know I'm doing the right thing. Women go through this in all kinds of abusive relationships. A parade of questions. It's another assault. I still struggle with my own probing. How could I let this happen to me?

Most importantly, I remember when my therapist asked, "So, do you want to know?" To which I replied, "Know what?" She said, "If you're a narcissist?" I had been called one so many times, I wondered if it were true. She knew it was eating at me, although I never said it (that's why she's amazing at her job). I agreed to hear from the expert. She said, "No! You don't have any signs of narcissism. But you question if you do because you've been gaslit for years, so I'm here to clear the air as your professional guide." She got it, she understood why I was so fearful of seeking therapy to begin with. I had been gaslit into believing *I* was actually the narcissist. That I was the problem. She often reminds me in moments of anxiety that I am not disordered. It's really refreshing to have a professional know me so well, to know my fears, yet objectively evaluate me with honesty.

Think of the gravity of someone breaking your confidence down to the point where you don't know who you are. In your thirties, you're supposed to know who you are. Most of the time, I know, and then I get lost sometimes. There were eight years of feeling lost. It's currently five years out, and it's a long road to recovery. This is the kind of abuse they say no one can see. It's internal. Internally, we have so many layers. It's up to us to keep all of them intact.

Identity is holistic. Retain it as your truth! This is extremely difficult to do when you are entangled in someone else's distortions. The more you practice self-care, the more you minimize the risk of entangling yourself. I can't stress this enough.

I remember times when all my accomplishments in residency and prior were overshadowed by my broken partner's lies and allegations. An administrator even joked to others I worked with that I might be sleeping with men in the office after hours. I'll never know if this joke was rooted in hearing these rumors about me that he spread or pure ignorance, but it stemmed from somewhere not based in fact. It's much easier to tarnish a female's reputation than a male's. He knew it would work.

With this utter breakdown of identity, you can't ignore the fact that there has to be a recovery process after something like this. Females could easily jump into another relationship that is similar. If you are not aware of what's happened to you or the type of person he was, it's extremely easy to fall for it again. If you don't get help, you assume blame, and then you find someone else. Not all relationships end this bad, but *all* narcissistic relationships are detrimental to your self-worth over time. You could stay that way if you don't realize what's happening to you and don't get help.

CHAPTER 11
Reclaiming Your Power

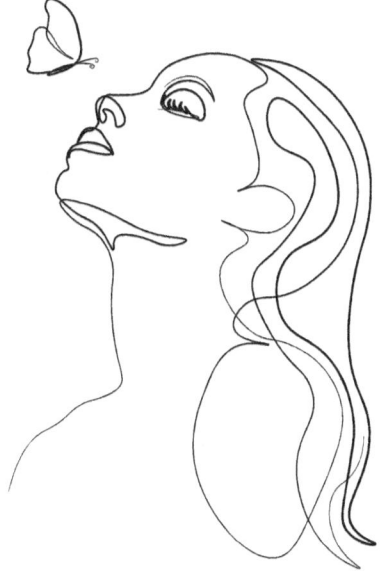

"Every crisis offers you extra desired power."

—William Moulton Marston

Power is the mother of all constructs when it comes to relationships. This is quite simply because relationships are not supposed to be about power—unless you are in a consensual S/M-type relationship. However, if you are powerful in yourself, you should covet and protect your power, which often requires boundaries. I will give you the perfect example.

My ex's relationships are plastered all over social media. Sometimes it cannot be helped as a doc-entrepreneur to run into news on these platforms, but this type of information does not affect me. However, as I mentioned before, three of his past girlfriends contacted me inquiring about domestic violence. In one case, he got physical, and she left instantly. The others did not. It is clear he has escalated. There will be other women.

When I receive messages from these women looking for help, it's a roller coaster for someone like me. Part of me wants to help, caution them, and they will see the pattern and escape. My therapist has warned me that is trying to save an earlier version of myself, and not effective. As I've said before, we are all on our own journey and have free will to decide what to do in every situation. If another woman stays, it is not my responsibility. Releasing responsibility for other people's actions that we know will harm them is tough for someone called to a healing specialty. The hardest was releasing responsibility for even his potential suicide. Not engaging with other people's choices is one of the ultimate self-care practices. It's a part of setting healthy boundaries and staying out of others' chaos.

This is power.

I have to keep myself very grounded when I hear stories of others being abused and manipulated. Old me would have wanted to help with my knowledge, but most people need a trained therapist, not just someone who has experienced it. It's also detrimental to my personal growth to stay in a mental space that I chose to leave long ago. We don't need to save everyone. It's one of the main reasons I felt called to write a book as a way to help others heal. I could help millions but not be on the individual energetics of every singular person's situation. We all have to protect ourselves. We all have to choose to save ourselves.

Thank god for therapists! Mine has made me so aware of the psychology of what is happening, and I know what to expect for the rest of my life. I am not surprised by anything, but I am so okay in my life, I know these actions—even so many years later—is a result of their world of dissatisfaction, their choices and projection to make someone else hurt with them. When that clicked, everything felt so impersonal. I have an impersonal view of my ex and others like him.

I'm currently entranced by my own life. I can observe it from a bird's eye view. In these relationships, they groom you so much to try to believe what is not true about yourself. Once I became confident again in who I was, all else literally became a lie. Getting to know yourself is not easy. It takes a lot of self-reflection and accepting that you accepted this behavior from someone. I see myself as someone that I never took the chance to fully know before. I almost have to check in to be sure this is me. The first thirty years of my life was a different story. I feel so powerful in myself now and not from a place of arrogance or hyper-protection. My happiness is the biggest shield from all this negativity. I don't recognize that person who was me six, seven years ago. For people like my ex, it's all pure reaction, need, instant gratification.

Today, I calculate. I discern. Is this in alignment with who I am today?

Karla just got out of another bad relationship. It's so common.

She repeated cycles. He had multiple girls throughout the relationships. With me being so open, she is finally asking herself how she is choosing these men. I couldn't see who Paul was. Giving people permission to ask themselves what they are not seeing feels good. Talk about relationships. Keep friends informed of questionable things or times that are making you uncomfortable, not just the good and shiny.

Human beings are here for love and belonging. You don't want to believe what you are experiencing or seeing when it's abuse. Believe it! Your safety and security are paramount, not romance, romantic impressions or romanticized versions of your situation. Fantasies or idealizing and minimizing what you are experiencing can make imprints forever. Let me give you an example.

With the U.S. political climate and handling of COVID-19 in 2020 and going into 2021, narcissism was at the root of a world leader's pathology. The entire country underwent abuse from a narcissist, and people were in different stages of this relationship: in love, confused, rejected, anxious, threatened. In addition to this, domestic violence and being cooped up with abusers in individual households compounded the issue for those in violent home situations. Racism was also rooted in this narcissism, with the entire Black community gaslighted and minimized systemically and overtly by some. This was also the case with how immigration was treated, enforcing supremacy and punishment of those that don't fit without giving any solid solution.

I'm sorry to say, but I feel strongly that we were all in a collective abusive relationship. And this is because a white man of power (like my ex) was able to play his cards to get ahead and blame others for his shortcomings, at any and all costs. I felt retraumatized hearing the rhetoric, gaslighting and blame shifting occurring on the news daily. I found it's really hard to discuss this with anyone who isn't aware what a narcissist is or looks like, because they are very charming and convincing humans. I isolated myself as much as I could, but my physical reaction and nausea to even hearing his voice was evident. Let me just state for the record, even if I had agreed with all views and policies, being retraumatized came from a visceral place, psychological maturity based on previous experience—not politics. Though the political position that holds such massive power over others opens the door to endless "supply" for the narcissist.

There is something that happens when you pay attention to your intuition and how you feel in your body when a disordered person is near physically or speaking. When you survive abuse, you are forever a hyper-aware, intuitive human. We are all intuitive, it's our survival skill, but not everyone has had to tune into it for actual survival in this day and age. When I am around someone who is disordered or perceived as dangerous to myself, I feel nauseated, frozen, and my breathing is shallower.

As a physician, the gaslighting specifically on healthcare workers and blame shifting for the pandemic handling, accusations of doctors profiting off of the pandemic and lack of consideration for death in general all made me feel sick as a dog. It hit me at some point, that we have all been exposed to narcissistic abuse on a global scale via our former administration. It made me even more aware that this topic of narcissistic abuse is as timely as ever. Lots of people noticed something was wrong, but I am one who could define it. This comes full circle to spirituality in my personal healing, and the collective need for society to heal from the daily abuse we don't even realize we're susceptible to. Healing can only occur with acknowledgement and acceptance of our own part in the process.

Domestic violence reports increased in 2020. When Joanne was getting death threats in text form, police stations flat out told her, "We are not staffed for this. We don't have the bandwidth to handle these cases. Unless you have been stabbed, know that you must protect yourself." She struggled with having things done appropriately in comparison to the collective voice of domestic violence, which is a long, running narrative of visible physical abuse only.

In the spirit of this book to offer solutions, as the Inter-American Commission on Human Rights and the United Nations have emphasized, countries must incorporate a gender perspective in their responses post-COVID-19. Several countries and nongovernmental organizations (NGOs) have already taken innovative steps in this direction. New campaigns also use social media to spread awareness of resources available to survivors, including hotlines, text message–based reporting, and mobile applications. Social distancing has increased people's reliance on technology and changed the way mental health, legal, and other social services are provided to survivors unable to leave their homes. With disruptions to the criminal justice system, countries have shifted to virtual court hearings, facilitated online methods for obtaining protection orders, and communicated their intentions to continue to provide legal protection to survivors.

What has been massively underestimated by a lot of individuals in this country during this time is the level of survival mode as animals we've been in from a biological standpoint. Everyone deals with this differently, but survival is not pretty. It's probable that people who have a history of violence will default in stressful situations. We have an individual threat everywhere we could potentially be.

For us women, and professional women, who have been secure in other areas of our identity, we don't view ourselves as trauma survivors. But saying I am a survivor is a flag that I wave now because it lets people know it's okay to share and they are not alone.

I've had to put up a lot of boundaries for various reasons. It speaks to the therapy of learning boundaries. It is apparent when

I need to place a boundary and it is never easy, but it's protection. I'm big on boundaries whenever I can sense a threat—and this threat can be raised by friends, that they are not respecting your time or limitations. If a relationship has a toxic dynamic, then a boundary is perceived as an attack. Someone who is healthy will perceive the boundary as time that you need or a space you are in. The reaction tells you a lot. If the reaction is that you are doing something *to* them, your boundary probably needs to be widened actually!

The fact that I was retraumatized speaks to the evidence of need for self-care. The continuous need. Once you have been abused, those things will show up in other arenas that you will not anticipate or expect. Trust me. I'm a doctor! It was once my story. This is everyone's story. Depression or feeling crazy or judging yourself. I'm elated to report that my story now includes true love and recent engagement!

All this trauma broke me out of so many cycles, as deeply rooted as childhood and later in the workplace. It has been so lifechanging and so positive. I know myself and I love myself.

Knowing yourself inside out before letting a new partner in is critical.

The average age of people who initially get into abusive relationships is in the 18-24 range. There's a reason I was 22 when I met my ex, and a reason he picked a 22-year-old after me; he learned from me that this age is naïve to his manipulation. They always go younger the second time. They learn how the first time (me). I feel fortunate that although I lost myself, and I put up with and made excuses for more than I want to admit, deep down, I knew it wouldn't be forever. I just didn't know how it would end. I used to think I was a strong person because of my education, athletics, and ability to multitask. I thought that meant all the strength I needed.

I have a new theory on strength these days. Someone like myself that others view as strong because of surviving something horrific doesn't actually feel strong. Being strong means you've been at your absolute lowest, weakest point in life; that feels awful. I felt weak, not strong. But I'm viewed as strong. On the day of my residency graduation I had just moved out of the house a few days prior. Some of the residents gave little individual speeches about those of us graduating. The girl that talked about me made her entire speech about how strong of a person I was, physically and mentally. I think she knew the gist of what was happening those few weeks but not explicit details. I remember sitting there, face broken out, hair thinning with patches of hair loss, exhausted eyes, makeup to cover my swollen, crying eyes, thinking, *she has the wrong person. I'm a mess. I'm not strong.* It meant a lot what she said that I was viewed that way, but in the moment, I felt like a fraud. I had just left an abusive fiancé, who had just been released from a mental institution. What strength? Now I know I am a very strong person. I know I'm resilient. But no one says they are "so happy this thing happened" to be that way. It's hard to thank bad situations even though you come out 1000x a more powerful person on the other side.

All that to say that ages 22-30 was a *huge* growing period. I'm thankful for these lessons I learned, and I know I'll never fall for it again. At 22, I was a bright-eyed first-year medical student who felt like she can take on the world, in a very naive way. At 30, I hit rock bottom, as I graduated residency a board certified physician. And now, at 35, I realize taking on the world is a much easier thing to do when you know yourself inside-out instead of listening to someone else make you into what they want you to be. I have found my energetic match is the best way to describe it. There is hope for every single survivor out there, that you do deserve someone great, because you yourself are great. My therapist always said a narcissist chooses the brightest lights to attach to. It is not because we are weak that we were targeted; in fact, it's our strength they want. They attach to that which they don't possess themselves. This keeps my confidence high on days I need to remind myself who in the world I am.

I live by resilience and balance today. What have I learned about myself? My intuition is usually right, and I shouldn't ignore it. I also learned that it was because I was a strong, independent yet empathetic person that I am a target for those that lack this, such as narcissists. I've learned that I really am capable of anything, and my doubts and fears were engrained in my head by outsiders and not my own beliefs. Relearning this has been the biggest breakthrough over the years.

I also solidified that I was put here to help others, and the things that happened to me only strengthened my mission and calling. They didn't happen to me, but for me. I wouldn't be who I am without these horrible experiences, so I am no longer embarrassed like I once felt. An easy life wouldn't have pushed me to fall this hard and force me to get up day by day even when I felt lifeless. My experience was simply an opportunity to show my inherent strength, not the thing that gave me strength. I want to make that distinction. This happened for me, not to me, but I had the means all along.

Trust your intuition over what someone is telling or showing you. Your gut feeling is usually right.

Never be afraid to seek therapy. Therapy is essentially a navigation through your past and present self. I'm more convinced those that face their struggles keep them from being stuck in old ways. We tend to accept we are a certain way because our parents were or some other situation, but you can always change. You aren't bound to your past. The results from therapy are worth the difficulty of facing the hard stuff—I could compare this to dieting in a lot of ways!

You are the only person holding yourself back from what you want. Nothing is forever or has to be. No matter how deep you think you are into someone else's world, you can always make the decision to leave if it isn't serving you, but it may be the hardest thing you will ever do.

Do regular audits of your relationships, your routines, and desires. Always ask yourself if what you're doing now is getting you somewhere or if it's draining you without reward.

You never have to apologize for being who you are or need to be when dealing with circumstances or eliminating bad people from your life. In fact, you must do this to prevent being held back. It's necessary to have boundaries. It doesn't make you a bad person for knowing what serves you and what doesn't. If you need space, take it.

When you're first out of a bad situation, simply sit still. Slowly find small routines, listen to your body. If you're tired, sleep. Eat well. Have some form of escape. Being alone is paramount for healing. Solitude is encouraged to get back in touch with yourself. Write down things you used to enjoy doing prior to the relationship, remind yourself of who you were before, and seek out those things a little at a time. Come back to you.

REFERENCES

Interviews by Author

Weatherly Camacho. Phone interview. June 26, 2018.

"Karla." Phone interview. July 2, 2018.

Diana Guy. Phone interview. July 25, 2018.

"Dawn." Phone interview. July 9, 2018.

"Joanne." Phone interview. February 12, 2021.

Publications

Anderson, Pauline. "Physicians Experience Highest Suicide Rate of Any Profession." *Medscape.* May 7, 2018. https://www.medscape.com/viewarticle/896257?src=soc_fb_180526_mscpedt_news_mdscp_suicide&faf=1

Bettinger-Lopez, Caroline, and Alexandra Bro. "A Double Pandemic: Domestic Violence in the Age of COVID-19." *Council on Foreign Relations.* May 13, 2020. https://www.cfr.org/in-brief/double-pandemic-domestic-violence-age-covid-19

CBS News. "Ohio State football coach Urban Meyer placed on leave amid claims he knew of abuse." August 2, 2018.

https://www.cbsnews.com/amp/news/ohio-state-urban-meyer-football-coach-administrative-leave-wednesday-after-zach-smith-fired-last-week/#app

Dykstra, Chloe. "Rose-Colored Glasses: A Confession." *Medium.* June 14, 2018. *https://medium.com/@skydart/rose-colored-glasses-6be0594970ca*

Psych Central. "How to Survive When Quarantined with a Narcissist." April 16, 2020. *https://psychcentral.com/pro/exhausted-woman/2020/04/how-to-thrive-when-quarantined-with-a-narcissist#3*

RAINN. "Victims of Sexual Violence: Statistics." *https://www.rainn.org/statistics/victims-sexual-violence*

Traverse Legal. "What is Defamation, Libel, and Slander?" https://www.traverselegal.com/defamation-libel-slander/#clip=2e7f1ot0gvdw

Wible, MD, Pamela. "Doctor revived after suicide tells all." *Kevin MD.* February 18, 2017. *https://www.kevinmd.com/blog/2017/02/doctors-revived-suicide-tells.html*

ABOUT THE AUTHOR

Danielle DonDiego, DO, MBA is a doctor, athlete, survivor, and self-care advocate. Board Certified in both Family Medicine and Obesity Medicine, she works with professional clients to evaluate and implement self-care practices so they can show up their best in life. She also works with patients via telemedicine with SteadyMD.com to educate and treat various chronic medical conditions. *Self-Care Rx* is her debut as an author.

www.ingramcontent.com/pod-product-compliance
Lightning Source LLC
Chambersburg PA
CBHW020910080526
44589CB00011B/529